2ω

Health, Happiness & Destiny
Come from Wise Choices

D1571277

Follow Me to a Better Life!

Richard Ruhling, MD, MPH

Hundreds of years ago, scribes copied the books of the Bible as a service to humanity and they did not copyright their work. This information is considered so important that everyone should be aware of its message and if the reader wants to copy it to share, that's fine. Please don't change the message nor charge more than a nominal price for expenses. Efforts were made to secure ok for graphic use and The "Fair Use" of a few is invoked for educational purposes by Total Health, a non-profit organization. Thank you for helping, May God bless you! ~RR~

Contents

A Tale of Two Cities

Charles Dickens' *Tale of Two Cities* says, "It was the best of times, it was the worst of times."

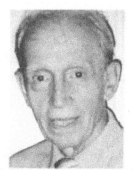

Salvatore Frascinella at 92,

It was so for Salvatore Frascinella, a 65-year-old NYC executive. His three cardiologists said he was too risky for bypass surgery, so they had him taking 12 pills a day, but he was getting worse-- he couldn't walk two blocks without severe chest pain--it was the worst of times.

But then he came to a health program that changed his life. One of his doctors said, If you quit the medicine, you'll die, but he lived another 30 years to age 95 with a return to tennis and the best of times!

In that account, we can see a *Tale of Two Destinies*-- we may die suddenly, and we discuss this later, or we might end life in a nursing home with an average of 9-13 prescriptions, some if needed for pain or sleep, others are daily, but these poor folks are so spaced out that they can stand in the hallway, staring into space as they fill their diaper, unaware of what's happening.

Susie Iwawaki, a friend of my wife, begged us to get her out of the nursing home. She was talking a dozen pills a day. Her blood sugars ran 200-300 and her mind was out of touch with reality-- we wheeled her into our home in a wheel chair. Stopping her drugs, she got better over 2-3 weeks--blood sugars are more than 100 points better--she walks and talks normally now.

Dr. Ken Cooper got America jogging with his book, *Aerobics*. His mother in her 90's went for some exercise on Friday, but didn't feel well over the weekend and she died on Monday. She didn't need any custodial care -- So much better than a nursing home. The pursuit of a better health destiny is essential to a good ending!

At 77 I enjoy better health than when I was 35 and didn't know the cause of my headaches that I'll explain in the chapter on food allergies.

In the past 60 years since college when I changed my diet, I've taken a prescription twice--once for intestinal flu when on a trip and didn't want to stop at every gas station, and once for a dental abscess, but I discovered that a clove of garlic next to the abscess also worked for pain.

One of my teachers in med school died last year at 104. He drove 50 miles a day to assist in heart surgery until he was 95!

This was at Loma Linda, a community featured in the *National Geographic* cover story on longevity as the only "Blue Zone" for health in North America. (November, 2005)

National Institutes of Health funded Loma Linda University $40 million to learn why the community lived an average of 7 years longer than other non-smokers. It was because of the writings of Loma Linda's founder, now in public domain and they are included in the mid-portion of this book.

If we stop to think, our bodies are made up from what we put in them from birth. The good news is that it's reversible. If we have a problem, we can change and the body starts getting better.

This principle applies to the mental, social and spiritual areas. Cutting TV and popular media and taking time for good inputs can reward us with happiness and a better destiny.

"What things are true, honest, lovely, good report...think on those things." Philippians 4:8.

Health Laws?

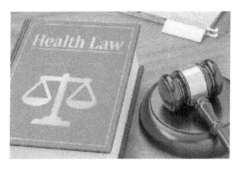

Laws of physics put men on the moon. We almost worship science for what it can do, but it must work in harmony with the laws of physics.

When it comes to health, some people think they can take a trip to the moon in a space capsule that their MD gives them. It spaces them out--we should beware of anything that alters mental function.

Computer programmers know that if it's "Garbage In," it's also "Garbage Out!" And that's true for the most wonderful computer of all, the human mind.

Most people dump 'garbage' into their minds and bodies so it's no surprise when some people start acting out what they see in movies or TV or video games as they go to malls or churches and begin shooting.

Many of them have been on mind-altering drugs, but we start with the basics.

Dr. Lester Breslow, Dean of UCLA, found 7 simple health habits were good for a 30-year advantage for people like Salvatore who kept the rules, compared to people who broke the rules like smoking, drinking and obesity. Here's *real* healthcare from Breslow--

Regular meals, no snacks

Daily breakfast

Moderate exercise, 2—3 times/week

Drinking 5 glasses of water a day

7—8 hours sleep/night

No Smoking

Not overweight

No alcohol, or moderate use

They answered yes to "Are you happy?"

Note: No specific foods were banned--Breslow began his study before the Framingham study of cholesterol ended its funding in 1968. If one follows a low fat, low cholesterol diet, there's huge benefit!

While teaching Health Science at Loma Linda University, I attended the American College of Cardiology Convention and heard Nathan Pritikin report the results of his diet and exercise program.

He showed how to reverse cardiovascular disease with a low-fat, low cholesterol diet. This included getting 85% of patients off of their drugs for high blood pressure and diabetes.

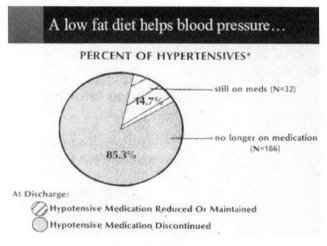

A low fat diet helps blood pressure...

PERCENT OF HYPERTENSIVES*

14.7% — still on meds (N=32)

85.3% — no longer on medication (N=186)

At Discharge:
Hypotensive Medication Reduced Or Maintained
Hypotensive Medication Discontinued

We might wonder how or why, but nearly half the calories in the diet of most Americans come from fat and it makes the blood sticky so more pressure is needed to circulate the blood and the cells stick together, like a roll of coins, absorbing less oxygen. Looking through a microscope, here's what it looks like....

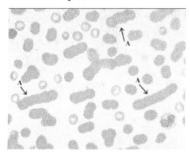

But when the those red blood cells stick together, they don't pick up oxygen in the lungs well, and the person can have chest pain called angina that limits their activity like Salvatore (above).

Fat also blocks insulin from taking glucose into the cell so the blood sugar goes up--diabetes! The average America gets nearly half his calories from fat. Think of the lettuce and tomato salad--it's only 20 calories? But with a dip of dressing, it's 120 calories, from the oil in the dressing!

It takes 12 ears of corn to make a tablespoon of corn oil for the dressing. We wouldn't eat 12 ears of corn at a meal, but we get the calories from them. This is why Dr. Colin Campbell, Prof. of Nutrition at Cornell is using the term, "whole food, plant-based." When we eat pastry, the shortening is fat, and not "whole food." Salads can become ok with chickpeas or pop corn, etc.

Hippocrates was right-- "Let your food be your medicine!" Sadly, the American Heart Association, the American Diabetic Association, the American Medical Association and mainstream media did NOTHING to help Pritikin--it wouldn't help them make money...they stand condemned for accepting drug money from drug companies to cooperate with bad science as will be explained later...

7

Heart Disease

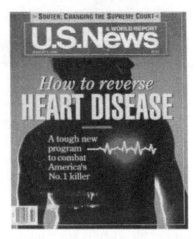

US News & World Report cover story in August, 1990 featured Dr. Dean Ornish who got his information from Pritikin--I think Pritikin was a light to many. Cleveland Clinic cardiologist, Dr. Caldwell Esselstyn makes some powerful statements about patients with heart disease making choices like Salvatore at the beginning of this book so they take control of their own healthcare. A link to his videos is at the end of this book.

And the foods that help reverse heart disease are good for the body in general. Cancer, diabetes and many chronic degenerative diseases are found less often in those eating a diet that's low in fat and cholesterol.

I grew up frying my own eggs and hamburgers and finishing off a half-gallon of ice cream while watching TV, but in college, I became a vegetarian and ice cream became a thing of the past.

The penicillin shots I got every other winter ended when I changed my diet and in the past 60 years, I've taken 2 or 3 pills for intestinal flu on a trip and similar for dental abscess pain until I found a clove of garlic also worked well for the gum boil.

Going on 78 and jogging up a gentle hill behind our house brings one to an appreciation of health that doesn't come from drugs.

Cancer

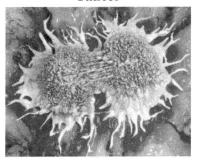

Cancer is next after heart disease as a leading cause of death. Cancer is related to lifestyle.

Bronchogenic carcinoma is strongly related to smoking. Breast cancer has hormonal and dietary influences, with less cancer since women stopped using hormones after menopause. Colon cancer has a dietary link to red meat and lack of fiber leading to constipation. Cancer of the pancreas has been linked to coffee as seen in the lead article of the *New England Journal of Medicine* for March 12, 1981. (Google or click here to see.)

The use of hormones, antibiotics, feeding of manure and rotten potatoes, (a contractor told me he built a loader for trucks to dump their load of rotten potatoes [costing only 1 cent/pound] and they would run down "like green snot" to mix with the cattle feed for protein. Now they also use manure. Slaughtering methods and "inspection" methods also spell disaster. "[A] federal meat inspector has all of 12 seconds in which to examine each beast [cattle], inside and out, as it passes by." *Wall Street Journal.*

The reporter assures us, "Not to worry: The U.S. Department of Agriculture has installed a long mirror so its inspectors...can glance at the back-sides of the dead cattle for abscesses, grubs and other parasites... Have you ever tried to see anything in a mirror 15 feet away through steam and fog?" asked inspector Michael Anderson. "You just hope that what you may have missed wasn't major."

9

Slaughtering standards allow removal of a cancer with the remainder of the carcass to be sold for human consumption. Those who understand how cancer spreads will know the dangers. For more insight, see "Flesh as Food" in a later chapter.

"The evidence that cancer can be prevented is now overwhelming. We should be able to reduce age-specific cancer incidence rates by 80— 90%" *NY State Journal of Medicine*, Aug. 1980, page 1401."

"[The] risk for developing cancer can be increased by as much as 10 times depending on diet. To minimize the risk of cancer, fresh fruits and vegetables and whole grain cereal products should be stressed...use of animal products should be de-emphasized." Dr. Colin Campbell, Cornell University. He reviewed thousands of scientific papers for the National Academy of Sciences panel on diet and cancer and he did the China Study. His videos are linked at the end of the book.

We are still waiting for the 10-fold benefits because we are still eating as we please and hoping it won't happen to us. We think medical science will find a cure. (Don't hold your breath!)

Early detection of cancer is important, but physical exams are not usually helpful. I examined executives for four years at Loma Linda University and had people who already knew they had a problem and also one man with a cancer that was not detected. His exam and urine were negative but a few months later, he passed some blood in his urine and had a kidney removed for cancer. My advice fits with the American Cancer Society in recommending the seven warning signs:

1. Unexplained lumps or bumps (as in breast, neck or arm pit).

2. Unexplained weight loss (20+pounds in a short time)

3. Unexplained passing of blood in bowels, urine, vagina, coughing.

4. Unexplained constipation (in spite of high fiber diet)

5. Unexplained or persistent hoarseness, beyond 2-weeks

6. A change in a brown mole.

7. A sore that does not heal.

Any lump or condition you have had for years without significant change would not be cancer. If you do have a question regarding one of the above, seek the best and most honest nonsurgical physician you can find. Ask questions and encourage his frankness with you. If it's malignant, ask him who in the closest metropolitan area, is the best surgeon he could recommend—the one he would go to. Go to that surgeon and again encourage frankness, but let him do the surgery as he would if he were the one who had the tumor—tell him to get it all, even if it means some disability on your part. The Bible says, "if your hand offend you, cut it off."

It is best to get rid of as much cancer as surgically possible and then adopt a vegan type of diet that is high in the protective foods, vitamins A,C,E, phytochemicals and fiber that seem to help the body's natural defenses. This would include more raw foods, nuts, seeds, sprouts, green drinks made with dark green leafy vegetables like kale. More on this and other habits later.

In medicine there seem to be exceptions to most rules, but I would probably not want to take radiation treatments unless I felt confident of significant benefit from a localized use. I am almost sure that I could not be persuaded to take chemotherapy, even though they may cite benefits. Chemotherapy is designed to poison the tumor but it also poisons your healthy cells (though hopefully not as much). Drugs tend to weaken your system and they all (even aspirin, Advil, and Tylenol) have adverse effects.

If you have surgery to remove the cancer, you may expect to feel good again, but you are not "out of the woods" for 3—5 years. If no recurrence by then, you may consider yourself cured. That's how medical science looks at it, by 5-year survival rates. If you do have a recurrence, I would be less inclined to trust medical science the second time—if they didn't get it all the first time, there is less of a chance now, and it's time to be very serious about the diet.

Please consider getting this dvd. It's an excellent tool to show how most diseases can be reversed by better eating habits. You can watch 8 minutes of it (88 minutes long, this 3rd edition is translated into other languages). You can see it and get it for just $10 <u>with a bonus book</u> at http://richardruhling.com/donate.aspx

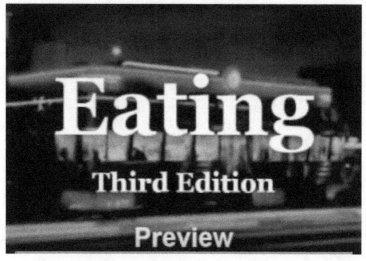

Eating is the #1 cause of disease, disability and death worldwide. Click the above link to see 8 minutes and donate $10 for the dvd that you will want to share with others. It includes a focus on cancer with Dr. Ruth Heidrich whose cancer had spread, but she refused the advice of five doctors, changed her diet and has a great testimony 20 years later! http://richardruhling.com/donate.aspx

There are places that do very well with natural remedies and I would emphasize this approach as most likely to have benefit. Recent research offers hope from Germany. Stem cells may be helpful in select cases. http://CancerTutor.com is a good website and you might get a copy of Suzanne Somers' book, *Knockout,* subtitled "Interview with Doctors Who Are Curing Cancer."

Stroke

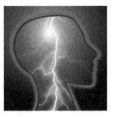

Stroke is the 3rd most common cause of death. High blood pressure is the major risk factor which can cause burst an artery in the brain, resulting in paralysis of arm or leg on one side, speech or all of this with coma, depending on severity.

The couple next to me on a plane related the example of their son who had a "massive stroke" at age 45, perhaps saved by their grandson, age 11 who called 911. They were praying for a miracle that their son, now unresponsive, would recover.

Yes, he had high blood pressure, but he didn't know the six or seven things he could do to lower his pressure.

#1. A high fat diet makes the blood sticky so it needs more pressure to circulate. Pritikin reported 85% of people taking blood pressure drugs no longer needed them on a low-fat diet…

A low fat diet helps blood pressure…

PERCENT OF HYPERTENSIVES*

14.7% — still on meds (N=32)

85.3% — no longer on medication (N=186)

At Discharge:

Hypotensive Medication Reduced Or Maintained

Hypotensive Medication Discontinued

#2. But it's not just oils or fats (like the shortening that goes into pastries) that makes blood pressure go up. Alcohol also makes the blood sticky.

#3. Caffeine makes the heart pump faster which also elevates blood pressure (coffee, tea & most soft drinks). The effect is short unless one drinks these beverages throughout the day.

#4. Loss of sleep makes stress hormones that also elevate blood pressure.

#5. Exercise neutralizes stress and lowers blood pressure, especially if it's an exercise that we like or don't dislike (stress).

#6. Salt makes us retain more fluid and also raises the blood pressure. Breaking these rules brings trouble, but the body forgives us if we repent and make better choices.

#7. Additional stroke factors include birth control pills or hormones, and eating just before bedtime. When we sleep, our blood is moving slowly, and fat in the meal can favor making mini-strokes, that set the stage for senility, etc.

Dr. Daniel Amen is a good source on brain health and he has videos linked at the back of this book.

Diabetes

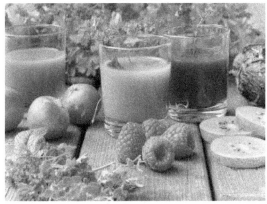

Next to cancer, diabetes is a most dreaded disease. It's the most common cause of blindness, kidney failure and amputation of a foot or lower leg. Patients often need dialysis or a kidney transplant in the US and they often die of heart attack or stroke.

Valmae Reed was an RN with Type I Diabetes. She got a kidney transplant from her sister and took 80 units of insulin a day, but reduced it to 18 units on a low fat, low cholesterol diet and exercise.

Most older folks are overweight when they get it, but sugar is not the main cause--it's high fat foods that block the insulin receptors in the cells.

Trained athletes tested diabetic after 3 days on a high fat diet. Similar story for Pima Indians that eat a high fat diet and commonly have diabetes.

Neal Barnard MD wrote the Program for Reversing Diabetes. His videos linked at the back of this book are excellent.

Allergies to Foods or Chemicals Can Cause Arthritis

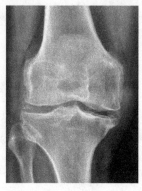

Doing Executive Health, I had several men tell me that sugar, cheese or meat bothered their joints. They were smart and had figured it out.

But when I got headaches, I couldn't see a relation to what I ate. At the university where I taught, I asked a neurologist if anything I ate or drank could be the cause. He assured me that food would be "a very rare cause" of my type of headache. I later learned that he didn't know!

When I went in practice with five other physicians, one was an allergist. Seeing people come hundreds of miles to see him, I asked how many of his patients with headaches he helped. He said about 90%! I asked him to test me. He did a cytotoxic test and listed several foods for me to avoid.

Long story short, the neurologist who taught medical students didn't know the cause of my headaches but the allergist discovered it was a food that I liked and ate regularly, but I would not have guessed it because the symptoms are delayed.

When a person becomes allergic to a food or chemical, the body builds up a tolerance to it and we get our symptoms on withdrawal, like smoking.

Even though tobacco is a poison, people don't get sick when they smoke--they get sick when they try to quit, on withdrawal. Foods can act as a stimulant and we get a high from them, but "what goes up must come down." When we get symptoms later, we usually don't make the connection to the cause.

Most physicians do not understand what these allergists know. And I have learned that there are a wide variety of medical conditions for which doctors prescribe symptomatic medication that can be caused by sensitivities to foods or chemicals.

If you have a chronic condition for which you or your physician have been unable to find a cause, do yourself a favor and change your diet completely for 10 days—like the 10 day trial of Daniel in the Bible. Eliminate all the things you usually eat and try rice with fresh fruits or vegetables that you don't usually eat, including some kind of bean or pea for protein. Don't use sugar, oil or margarine for the trial (corn syrup or oil is a common sensitivity). You might think you are dying, but the withdrawal gets better in a couple days.

Let me use my own experience to illustrate. On becoming a vegetarian, I learned to love whole wheat bread, sandwiches, cereals and granola. I was over-eating these and when a food is not properly digested, some long-chained proteins can be absorbed and act as an antigen (allergic factor).

Initially it's no problem, but in time, our load of antigens becomes heavy and we get symptoms, like the hay fever patient in pollen season.

With foods or chemicals, the symptoms are often related to withdrawal from the food, so that when we eat the food again, the symptoms may get less and we think we need it. It becomes a favorite food, with symptoms of unknown cause.

The following conditions are commonly caused by food or chemical sensitivities:

1. Headaches: tension, migraine and cluster types

2. Chronic fatigue, awaken un-refreshed

3. Muscle tension and tightness, especially in neck and shoulders

4. Hyperactivity in children, chronic nervousness in adults

17

5. Chronic sinusitis, nasal stuffiness

6. Chronic dizziness, vertigo, loss of balance

7. Chronic cough, wheezing or asthma which can have a food component. For example, dairy causes mucus production and in the lungs this causes wheezing. Eggs can also be an asthma factor.

8. Many if not most skin rashes

9. Chronic digestive problems, colitis, gas, cramps, diarrhea. More help on digestion in a later chapter

10. Bed wetting in children and urinary frequency in adults that can seem like prostate problems in men

11. Joint pains, swelling, fluid retention

12. Chronic anxiety, insomnia, depression or nervousness

13. Compulsive eating, overweight One of the following books may be of help, available in paperback, sometimes found in libraries or health food stores.

Dr. Burger's Immune Power Diet, Dr. Mandell's 5-Day Allergy Relief System, How to Control Your Allergies by Dr. Robert Foreman. It's been a few years…there may be more recent ones now.

If the reader has one of the above problems but is unable to sort out the cause, I would recommend a physician who is a member of the American Academy of Environmental Medicine.

These physicians are more intelligent regarding foods and chemicals than other doctors. If your symptoms from foods are severe and you aren't able to discover the cause by trying an elimination of foods as described above, you might want to call to find one practicing near you. Their headquarters is in Wichita, KS, 316 684 5500.

I can't vouch for the videos on food allergy, but there's a link at the end for some.

Alcohol

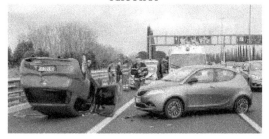

Accidents have been the fifth leading cause of death but they account for most deaths under 30. Alcohol and drugs are the cause in most accidental deaths at any age. Drugs are playing a bigger role now with the opioid overdoses.

Alcohol is estimated to be responsible for one third of accidental deaths. The Exxon Valdez reminds us that many of the tragic accidents by air, land and sea are due to alcohol.

Alcohol has ruined more marriages and business partnerships that any other single factor.

As the oldest drug in history, it should alert us to the fact that millions today take other mind-altering drugs that can also be responsible for accidents and terrorist acts as we see in the news, some are prescription drugs.

Studies show people worry about antidepressants that seem similar to illicit substances, or maybe they feel shame and keep their use secret, with fears of addiction, "going cold turkey," and the potential for personality changes—all of these and more may be involved in mind-altering medication.

Other studies show that more than two-thirds of people taking antidepressants do not actually meet the criteria for depressive disorders. Yet about 12 percent of the population from 12 up are taking them. When we consider the huge risk it involves, we should ignore the drug ads, "Ask your doctor" and maybe try some natural remedies like St. Johns Wort that is used often in Europe for depression.

Alcohol was a major factor in the fall of Babylon, Rome, France and Pearl Harbor in World War II. Alexander the Great conquered the world but was conquered by alcohol and died in his 30's. Most of those who drink to cope with stress sooner or later become alcoholic. One out of three teenagers has a problem with alcohol. Alcohol is a major factor in broken homes and ruined people.

Alcohol causes disability, disease and death. It figures in one third of suicides, half of murders and 2/3 of rapes and violent crimes. If a food caused even a few deaths, lawmakers would ban it, but Washington DC is the alcoholic capital of America with most politicians being "under the influences" directly or by its lobbyists.

Alcohol is the oldest of all drugs and a forerunner of tranquilizers. It is a leading cause of birth defects, mental retardation and "spontaneous abortion." It is heavily implicated in half the robberies, rapes, marital violence and child abuse.

One study reported 95% of criminals in California prisons are alcoholic or use alcohol in some form. A priest who killed someone while driving under the influence of alcohol told a seminar group that we hear much about the evils of tobacco, but it is only a pimple on the rear end of a giant, alcohol!

"With a liberal hand, God has bestowed His blessings upon men. If His gifts were wisely used, how little world would know of poverty or ruin! It is through the greed of gain and the lust of appetite that the grains and fruits given for our sustenance converted into poisons that bring misery and ruin...

"Millions upon millions of dollars are spent in buying wretchedness, poverty, disease, degradation, lust, crime, and death. Houses of prostitution, dens of vice, criminal courts, prisons, poorhouses, insane asylums, hospitals, all are to a great degree filled as a result of the liquor sell work." *The Ministry of Healing*, p 337, 338.

Blue Cross reported that drinking and smoking were the underlying factors responsible for the high cost of care which was more than three times greater than those whose medical records did not suggest drinking or smoking was a problem. I have been asked to indicate the cause of hospitalization as a nervous disorder, because otherwise insurance wouldn't pay!

Since "an ounce of prevention is worth a pound of cure," the following statement is worth considering: "In this fast age, the less exciting the food, the better...wrong habits of eating and drinking destroy the health and prepare the way for drunkenness." Ibid.

This statement was the basis for a university experiment. Rats on a "junk food" diet versus a vegetarian diet drank five times more alcohol than on the a vegetarian diet.

Coffee doubled the alcohol consumption and doubled again when spices were added.

One of the worst effects of alcohol is that it leads to other drug problems. Much more could be said because there are many problems associated with the use of alcohol, but experience shows that if the above is not sufficient, neither would a book be enough to change one's mind!

Alcoholics Anonymous is a good source of help with their 12 Steps that include God at the beginning. Sadly, some groups sit around and smoke while they talk about the evil of alcohol.

Caffeine's Deceptions

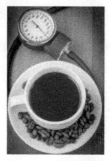

Caffeine is the most common yet unrecognized cause of health problems in America, as tea may be for the world. It's a major contributor to the high cost of medical care.

Companies that make their money from the addiction of others should be surcharged.

When something is good for the body (like, exercise), it benefits the body many ways, but when something is bad for the body (like caffeine), it is manifested in many problems. I have worked in emergency rooms or clinics that see a cross-section of this country's millions suffering symptoms from caffeine, but they don't see the cause.

1. Headaches: Tension, migraine and cluster types. Most physicians do not recognize caffeine to be the cause of headaches since many drug companies include caffeine as one of the ingredients to relieve the pain.

But the headache results from withdrawal just as smokers get symptoms when they try to quit. So coffee is prescribed for headaches the day after surgery; Anacin, Excedrin, APC, BC or Goody Powders, "cure" the headache, but maintain the addiction.

The same may be said for Cafergot or Fiorinal (sometimes prescribed for migraine). People need to be willing to break their destructive habits and pay the price of withdrawal. If they want health, they have to suffer through the pain (taking Tylenol or Advil temporarily is o.k.), stop all caffeinated pills or beverages, so that when the headache is gone, the addiction is broken and they have eliminated the most common cause of headaches! Birth control pills or hormones are also a common cause of headaches as any PDR (*Physician's Desk Reference* which most libraries have as a reference) will show.

2. Stomach troubles: Heartburn, gastritis, ulcers and hiatal hernia. Caffeine is one of the most powerful stimulants of gastric acid. Caffeine supports the antacid industry of Tums, Rolaids, Mylanta, and expensive drugs like Tagamet, Zantac, Pepcid, and Axid. Guidelines for these expensive drugs indicate they should not be used regularly except for 4—6 weeks to cure an ulcer, but millions use beverages, foods and analgesic drugs that irritate the stomach and take these drugs continuously, adding to a risk.

3. Sleep Disorders and Insomnia. Sleeping pills are big business, thanks to caffeine's effects of slower to sleep, shallow sleep and easy wakefulness. Many who don't think they have a problem find they sleep much better without it!

4. Nervous disorders: Millions of Americans are addicted to tranquilizers, and their need for nerve pills began with their addiction to caffeine which stimulates the nerves. Then they want something to calm them. A tragic cycle of foolishness that is easier to prevent than cure. Many caffeine users have anxiety—the most common cause for tranquilizers in America. Every day countless patients in doctors' offices are given Valium, Xanax, Ativan and other costly Rx' s to cope with nervous problems, with scarcely a thought that patients develop this need by using caffeine. Hyperventilation and panic attacks are seen daily in any emergency room. The cause is usually unknown, but questioning uncovers caffeine as a factor in most of these cases.

5. Cardiovascular problems: Caffeine speeds the heart rate and therefore raises the blood pressure. It causes abnormal beating (premature ventricular contractions) and lowers the threshold for ventricular fibrillation, a fatal arrhythmia if not defibrillated quickly. These are reasons why it is not allowed in coronary care units. It also elevates triglycerides (blood fat levels).

6. Cancer: The fourth leading cancer cause of death is pancreas and in a major study published in the *New England Journal*, caffeine had a strong correlation.

Bladder cancer in women was found to be 2.5 times more frequent in women who drank 2—3 cups of coffee per day. Colon cancer is also higher.

7. Birth defects: The most common defect (cleft palate or hare lip) is linked to caffeine. The Food and Drug Administration advises pregnant women to avoid all caffeine because of premature births and low birth weight. Animal studies show increased risk of birth defects.

8. Fibrocystic disease of the breast. Medical textbooks recognize the role of caffeine in causing this most common reason for breast surgery, mammograms. Fibrocystic disease is also a risk factor for breast cancer.

9. Blood Chemistry: Caffeine elevates blood sugar and probably catecholamine levels—excitement hormones.

10. Bad Habit Glue is what Dr. Pavlov, the famous Russian scientist called coffee. Most Americans could not wake up and face the day because their lifestyle is so abusive, but caffeine whips their nerves and they charge off to work in a state of stress that lasts all day.

Caffeine is also a major reason why smokers are unable to quit tobacco, because tobacco stimulates the nerves and the person needs a smoke to calm them. The 5-Day Plan to Stop Smoking has shown it is easier to quit both tobacco and caffeine, than to quit only smoking. After considering the evidence against caffeine, it is time to quit!

Tips on Quitting

1. Choose to be free. The brain is programmed to accomplish what we choose. If we choose to give up something that is against us, the creative powers of the mind will seek to accomplish it.

2. Substitute non-caffeinated beverages. Use cereal coffees like Postum, Pero and Breakfast Cup, and fruit juices instead of colas, and herb teas instead of Lipton. Try Tylenol or Advil for withdrawal headache or if severe, as a doctor for a prescription containing no caffeine.
3. Withdrawal migraines may be helped by use of a double sink with hot water in one side and cold in the other side. Put your forearms and hands in the hot for 3-5 minutes and then switch to cold for 1/2 to 1 minute. Repeat a couple times. This vascular exercise will reduce the severity of the headache.
4. Ask God for help. Choose to follow truth and right principles. Caffeine is a Drug: Say No to Drugs.

Dying to Smoke

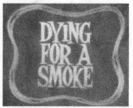

You Can Quit with This Strategy!

"There are just two keys to breaking an addiction and though they can help to quit any addiction, this article focuses on smoking for folks who are tired of smoker's breath, $6/pack and health problems. This strategy helped 100 people to quit in a 5-Day Plan at the University of AZ when I was training years ago.

The first key is the strength of the strategy one follows to quit. The 5-Day Plan has helped well over 30 million people to quit since it's beginning nearly 60 years ago. (Google) The success is due to its physiologic design (below) to minimize craving and withdrawal symptoms so that if a person follows the program, most people succeed.

The second key is the strength of commitment to quit. If a person is offered $1 million to quit, most people would find a way to do it, even if they had to be locked up 5 days!

Life and health are worth more than a million dollars. Smokers are slowly trading life and health for the pleasure of satisfying a self-inflicted addiction, a monkey on their back that they would gladly give it up if they knew how and at $6, a pack a day will cost them $100,000 in 40-some years!

The wasted money is not nearly so bad as the loss of health that 'healthcare' can't buy. Young men, average age of 26 who died suddenly in motor cycle accidents had their lungs studied under a microscope. They had bronchiolitis with fibrosis--changes that are seen in emphysema, a disease that comes years later, but early changes were seen in all of those who smoked!

The point is: changes are occurring, whether the smoker feels it or not, and the last months of life are spent in bed struggling to breathing oxygen through a tube where smoking is not allowed--the end is not good.

Most people told themselves when they started smoking, "If this gets to hurting me, I'll quit." It's time to do that because the hurt is a silent damage that one can't feel until it's often too late. A smoker has everything to gain by giving this their best effort.

There are other reasons, like doing it for spouse or to be an example for one's family. They say kissing a smoker is like kissing an ash tray. One of the best motives is religious belief or as Shakespeare said, "to thine own self be true."

Millions of smokers believe in God, but if they think God intended us to inhale smoke, He should have made our nose with a single opening and a stronger filtration system. God designed the body as a living temple for His Spirit that He gives to every person to guide them. If we tune in, we can know what's right.

The key to success in quitting is to keep the motives in mind and stay with the plan. Cutting down on cigarettes is like cutting the tail off a dog, one inch at a time. Tapering the habit does not work. The next cigarette is the whole habit. Quit "cold turkey."

The best time to quit may be a Thursday night so a person can tough it through Friday at work and not have to cope with stress of work on Saturday and Sunday. Beware of celebrating with alcohol or you are likely to blow smoke again.

The craving is physiologic, like the urge to go to the bathroom. If one says a decided No, the craving goes away for a while but returns like the need to go to the bathroom.

Having a strategy to stall it off is helpful. When urge to smoke comes, do the following--

1. Repeat your decision and commitment--"I choose to quit."
2. Take some slow deep breaths--hold it for a few seconds and exhale till you can't squeeze any more air out. Think of this as a lung exercise. The deep breathing helps cope with stress by a mechanism that we don't have space to explain here.

3. Get a drink of water. Think of it as washing nicotine out of your body. The sooner it's gone, the easier life will be for you.

4. Go for a short walk. If at work, go to the fountain or bathroom. If at home, around the block or to the mailbox is good. Dress warm and breathe deep.

5. The most important part of this program is this: Do NOT drink coffee, tea or colas! The caffeine excites nerves that will cry for a smoke to calm them. The caffeine and nicotine are both alkaloid neurotoxins that work in opposite directions to keep the smoker in balance. The caffeine will drive the person back to smoking. Headache can be due to caffeine withdrawal; take an aspirin or Tylenol, but not anything w caffeine.

6. To wake up without coffee, go to bed early. A warm tub bath helps to relax the nerves. Set your alarm a half hour earlier. Dress warm and go out for a brisk walk around the block. Then take a hot shower for 3 minutes and turn the hot water off for 15-30 seconds of cold. You won't have a heart attack and the lift you get will keep you alert all morning without any need of coffee or the let-down that comes with caffeine.

7. Alcohol is big risk #2. The smoker has to decide, which is more important and everything must align with the choice and decision to quit. Good motives should not be jeopardized by a bad decision for a cup of coffee or a beer. And once quit why go back to bad habits. Dr. Pavlov said coffee is "Bad Habit Glue!"

8. Just as alcohol affects the brain and willpower, there is a similar effect from a heavy meal. It draws blood from the brain to the stomach and smokers are used to having a smoke after a meal. They must break this pattern for the first few days of quitting.

Some physicians recommend fasting for the first day. Fasting intensifies will power and doing so allows maximum blood to the brain for clear thinking. Especially avoid high fat, high protein and a full stomach during these 5 days, eat less.

If a person does not want to fast, they can get an assortment of fruit juices to help the body detox and cleanse itself. This can be done with good results for day 1 and then light eating of fruit or juices for day 2 and 3 gets you over the hump.

Break the habit patterns. Sitting in same "smoking" chair is unwise. Go out for a walk in the fresh air after meals.

For years a cigarette has brought comfort like an old friend. Change that association by wearing a strong rubber band on the wrist and when the craving comes, give that rubber band a big snap so that the brain gets pain with the desire to smoke!

Whether or not you believe in God, ask Him to help you! Communists who don't believe in God have said, "God, if you exist, help me," and they have found help.

If a buddy or friend would support quitting, call for a chat when things are tough. Think of the next cigarette as the whole habit. It you don't smoke it, you will be free. Regarding habit, after time erase the 'h' and you still have a bit; more time and you still have it. Know your weakness--don't put yourself in harm's way.

If a person is used to a night out at the bar, finding a different way to celebrate and choosing some non-smoking friends to associate with is important.

Don't trade the smoking for eating every time the craving comes. Millions have quit without doing so. If you want something to do with your hands, open a pack of gum, or carry some lemon slices in a plastic bag for a few days--they cut the craving!

In summary so far, most medical problems are diseases of choice: what we choose to put in our mouths. If we choose wisely, we should not need medical care that is also a leading cause of death.

Surprise: the Leading Cause of Illness & Death!

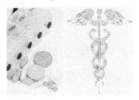

A key feature of longevity is the practice of self-health care rather than depending on medical care for prescription drugs. This is because Adverse Drug Reactions have made medical care a leading cause of death.

The definition of an adverse drug reaction is an unexpected reaction from a medicine "properly prescribed and administered." In other words, it wasn't malpractice. It was a good prescription for that condition, and it wasn't an overdose. The above article reported hospital data where a nurse dispensed the proper dose, but the patient, for some strange reason, reacted adversely.

Adverse Drug Reactions put 2.2 million people in hospitals and 106,000 died, "making these reactions between the fourth and sixth leading cause of death." *Journal of American Medical Assoc*, 4-15-1998

How many died at home? 199,000 according to the *Western Journal of Medicine*. June, 2000. Deaths in and outside hospitals from Rx totaled 305,000 then, with 8 million admissions to the hospital and 3 million for long-term care (nursing homes--these people were messed up for life!)

"From 1998 through 2005, reported serious adverse drug events increased 2.6-fold...fatal adverse drug events increased 2.7-fold." *Archives of Internal Medicine* Sep 10, 2007, p 1752.

But if deaths increased 2.7 fold from 1998 to 2005, by 2020 we might expect those deaths to increase 8-fold. Multiplying 305,000 deaths/year by 8, prescribed drugs killed 2.4 million people/year. Many are not old people in nursing homes--most of them weren't even in the hospital. 2.4 million deaths/year is 6,000 deaths--two 9/11's daily!

Confronted with these figures, a U.S. Senator said told me I was wasting my time, "they own us," referring to the pharmaceutical industry that spends millions per year on congressional re-election campaigns, says (Marcia Angell, MD, former editor of *New England Journal of Medicine* (*60 Minutes*' interview), now teaching at Harvard. These people are false to their oath of office.

What happens is unpredictable, and it happens more often than you hear about in the news that's sponsored by the drug companies.

I once relieved a doctor for a week in a pain clinic where everyone seemed addicted to hydrocodone or xanax. They were victims of poor prescribing by doctors who liked the gifts that drug companies gave for prescribing them.

When people hurt themselves by bending or heavy lifting the usual treatment is bed rest, moist heat and a muscle relaxant. But too often, they go back to work before the injury has had time to heal, and they feel great with the Rx until they try to quit it and they get their pain again.

So they become addicted to it, feeling the pain whenever they try to quit the medicine.

Chiropractic care is 1st choice in Europe for back injuries but in this country, the AMA is trying to force alternatives out of business. Chiropractors refer to MD's when they can't help, but it doesn't go the other way.

My wife, Norma, was in good health and as a chiropractor's daughter, she didn't believe in prescription drugs, but she got a bladder infection.

She got a prescription for Cipro, commonly used for urinary infection. Norma was better after only a few doses and she discontinued it. But a few months later she developed a rash. I recognized it as petechial hemorrhage and suggested she see her doctor.

He called back after a blood test to say he made an appointment for her the next morning at a hematologist. Long story short, her blood platelets that were supposed to be 100,000-200,000 were 20,000. Over the months that followed, she had a splenectomy and high doses of Prednisone, blood transfusions and gamma globulin.

Her platelets continued to drop and she developed a severe headache one evening and I had to help her back from the bathroom. She died of a stroke (brain hemorrhage.)

Her doctor signed the death certificate as Idiopathic Thrombocytopenic Purpura.

I was taught in my internal medicine residency that "idiopathic" meant idiotic on the part of the doctor for not knowing the cause, and pathetic on the part of the patient; that's "idiopathic" (unknown cause).

Looking up Norma's antibiotic—the only Rx medication she had taken during our 19 years of marriage, I discovered that Cipro (taken a few months before her trouble began) can affect the bone marrow and cause the platelet problem she had.

I agree with Dr. Carson that Obamacare, which forces medical care on people who may not want prescriptions or vaccinations, "is the worst thing since slavery."

You can see a YouTube, "government healthcare" that can fill you in...The drug companies had a key role in helping to write the Obamacare plan, We should have known...

Congress closed the door to alcohol ads on TV--alcohol is the oldest drug in history, but they have opened the door to modern drugs that are equally bad, and more deceptive.

It is interesting that in the Bible, Revelation 18:2-4 makes a call to come out of the confused systems that it calls Babylon, "for by her sorceries were all nations deceived," verse 24. The Greek word that's translated sorcery is *pharmakeia.*

The reference to "Babylon" reminds us of the "Tale of Two Cities" at the beginning of this book. In the end, we may be in Babylon--amid the confused systems of our time, needing a call out, or we may have a different destination that we will see later.

Sorcery may seem like a harsh word, but when a person takes a chemical that the body sees as a poison, yet relieves the symptoms, it may seem like sorcery or magic, but trouble comes sooner or later.

Drill's Textbook of Pharmacology in Medicine, Chapter 5, Mechanisms of Drug Action, offers this insight: "In the widest sense of the word, every drug is by defninition a poison. Pharmacology and toxicology are one, and the art of medicine is to use these poisons beneficially."

The reference to toxicology is an echo of how the 'science' of pharmacology developed when they saw half the lab rats die from a chemical. The percentage has changed, but life is a rat race as one MD said...

If a person's blood pressure is high, it might be ok to take a drug and get it down rather than have a stroke and be paralyzed, but wouldn't it be better to eat less grease or fried foods, less salt, stress, and get more exercise and sleep? All of these are choices we can make to lower blood pressure.

Vaccinations: Another example of how pharmacology is poison, is the use of mercury as a preservative in multi-dose vials of vaccine. They say the amount is small, but if they warn pregnant women not to eat tuna fish because of the mercury content, what do we think it will do to babies?

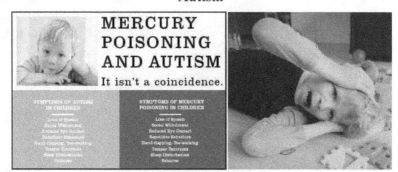

The symptoms of autism & mercury toxicity are the same: loss of speech, social withdrawal, reduced eye contact, repetitive behavior, hand-flapping, toe-walking, temper tantrums, sleep disturbances and seizures.

By 2 months of age, a baby gets a 2nd dose of Hepatitis B vaccine and SIX other shots--a total of 8, when their tiny systems cannot handle the mercury.

https://kidshealth.org/en/parents/med13m.html The result?

Japan has a much lower incidence of autism--they delay the vaccination process till after 1 year of age when the baby's immune system is more developed.

Why vaccinate? I reared six children with n0 vaccinations and they all grew up healthy. Mennonites and others that don't vaccinate have no autism. Here's a powerful 1-minute video on autism by pediatrician, Dr Mayer Eisenstein https://bit.ly/2knnIKI

This information on drugs and mercury fits well with what a favorite author, Ellen White, wrote 100 years ago, but let me first explain why she's great in my book.

She founded the school that I attended, but she didn't want drugs to be part of the curriculum. She wrote,

"A practice that is laying the foundation of a vast amount of disease and of even more serious evils is the free use of poisonous drugs. When attacked by disease, many will not take the trouble to search out the cause of their illness. Their chief anxiety is to rid themselves of pain and inconvenience. So they resort to patent nostrums, of whose real properties they know little, or they apply to a physician for some remedy to counteract the result of their misdoing, but with no thought of making a change in their unhealthful habits. If immediate benefit is not realized, another medicine is tried, and then another. Thus the evil continues.

"People need to be taught that drugs do not cure disease. It is true that they sometimes afford present relief, and the patient appears to recover as the result of their use; this is because nature has sufficient vital force to expel the poison and to correct the conditions that caused the disease. Health is recovered in spite of the drug. But in most cases the drug only changes* the form and location of the disease. Often the effect of the poison seems to be overcome for a time, but the results remain in the system and work great harm at some later period. [*This describes Adverse Drug Reactions!]

"By the use of poisonous drugs, many bring upon themselves lifelong illness, and many lives are lost that might be saved by the use of natural methods of healing.

The poisons contained in many so-called remedies create habits and appetites that mean ruin to both soul and body. Many of the popular nostrums called patent medicines, and even some of the drugs dispensed by physicians, act a part in laying the foundation of the liquor habit, the opium habit, the morphine habit, that are so terrible a curse to society.

"The only hope of better things is in the education of the people in right principles. Let physicians teach the people that restorative power is not in drugs, but in nature. Disease is an effort of nature to free the system from conditions that result from a violation of the laws of health. In case of sickness, the cause should be ascertained. Unhealthful conditions should be changed, wrong habits corrected. Then nature is to be assisted in her effort to expel impurities and to reestablish right conditions in the system.

Ellen White's inspiration to have a school to teach natural remedies was a century ahead of our times, and it's sad that church leaders did not respect her "no" to the teaching of pharmacology. They wanted Loma Linda to be accredited by the American Medical Association. Against her will, they voted it to become like other medical schools when they had light pointing to something better.

This was when the smartest people went to Battlecreek Hospital for natural treatment without drugs a century ago--they included people like CW Barron, Wm Jennings Bryan, Luther Burbank, Admiral Byrd, Dale Carnegie, Amelia Earhart, Thomas Edison, Harvey Firestone, Henry Ford, SS Kresge, Ivan Pavlov, JC Penny, CW Post, Eleanor Roosevelt, George Bernard Shaw, Upton Sinclair Wm Taft, Count Tolstoy, and more.

Nevertheless, the community of Loma Linda founded by Ellen White, was featured in the *National Geographic* cover story on longevity as the only "Blue Zone" for health in North America...

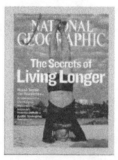

Further supporting the visionary writing of Ellen White, National Institutes of Health granted Loma Linda $40 million to learn why the community lived 7-11 years longer than other non-smokers.

Most of it has to do with her counsels on foods and eating habits that we excerpt from her book, *The Ministry of Healing,* published in 1905, now in public domain.

Let's not forget our choice of destiny--medical care is not how we want life to end. We can do better by making wise changes now.

A Better Weigh Without Dieting

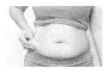

To summarize the best foods for health, we should consider whole foods that are plant-based that don't have lots of processing. As one doctor said, Don't read the labels--don't eat foods with labels on them!

We should minimize the use of oils and fats. Whole foods means that it's ok to eat olive or nuts, but don't use peanut butter and jelly for the sandwich! The sandwich can be good with a slice of tomato and toast with sliced banana isn't bad.

Green drinks as a salad with raw greens whizzed in a fruit juice is good nutrition, and throw in some alfalfa sprouts.

Make a deal with yourself to enjoy as much of those foods as you wish twice a day--breakfast and early afternoon, but do your best to fast each evening. That meal puts the weight on.

Just as the ground hog eats its last meal and hibernates for winter with a slow metabolism, our metabolism slows each night and food we've eaten after 3 or 4 is often stored in the form of fat.

Drink water and go for a walk! At first you'll miss the meal, but you'll soon be sleeping better to awaken more refreshed with a better appetite for breakfast, and doing so will save you from a fast break later in the morning.

Being rigid about meal times with nothing between will help toward your goal. To suppress appetite, a cup of hot water w a little lemon ~15 minutes before the meal. Much of what we interpret as hunger is thirst and every good weight-loss program recommends fluids. It's also an excellent aid to digestion.

Beware the starches? No, beware of what we put on them. High fat dressings or sauces will sabotage our goals. Use low-calorie dressings. If you do dairy, a low-fat cottage cheese or some peas or beans can make the salad more interesting, or try a diced apple.

Natural Remedies

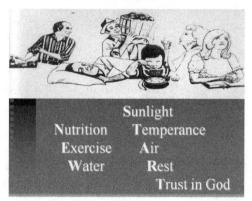

	Sunlight
Nutrition	Temperance
Exercise	Air
Water	Rest
	Trust in God

"Pure air, sunlight, abstemiousness, rest, exercise, proper diet, the use of water, trust in divine power--these are the true remedies. Every person should have a knowledge of nature's remedial agencies and how to apply them. It is essential both to understand the principles involved in the treatment of the sick and to have a practical training that will enable one rightly to use this knowledge." *The Ministry of Healing,* p 126,127.

The above statement is profound and I know health institutions that base their programs on those eight "remedies." The graphic above is from a painting on the wall of an institution where I worked 45 yrs ago.

A third of a century ago, Paul Harvey, News Columnist for the *Times Herald* wrote, "Once upon a time, 100 years ago, there lived a young lady named Ellen White. She was frail as a child, completed only grammar school, and no technical training, and yet she lived to write scores of articles and many books on the subject of healthful living.

"Remember, this was in the days when doctors were still bloodletting and performing surgery with unwashed hands. This was in an era of medical ignorance bordering on barbarism. Yet Ellen White wrote with such profound understanding on the subject of nutrition that all but two of the many principles she espoused have been scientifically established." August 24, 1960.

One of the two items not proven in 1960 was her statement on cancer found in her book. *The Ministry of Healing:* "Those who use flesh foods little know what they are eating. Often if they could see the animals when living and know the quality of the meat they eat, they would turn from it with loathing. People are continually eating flesh that is filled with tuberculous and cancerous germs. Tuberculosis, cancer, and other fatal diseases are thus communicated." p 313.

https://bit.ly/2lySOQ4 This is now supported by news reports such as this, https://nbcnews.to/2lySLDS

NEW START (see graphic above for acronym)

These remedies are treated in greater depth in the book, *The Ministry of Healing.* The author received a six-page review by Dr. Clive McCay: Professor of Nutrition, Cornell Univ, New York

Excerpting his review--"Every modern specialist in nutrition whose life is dedicated to human welfare must be impressed in four respects by the writings and leadership of Ellen G. White.

"In the first place, her basic concepts about the relation between diet an health have been verified to an unusual degree by scientific advances of the past decades...

"In the second place, everyone who attempts to teach nutrition can hardly conceive of a leadership such as that of Mrs. White that was able to induce a substantial number of people to improve their diets.

"In the third place, one can only speculate about the large number sufferers during the past century which could have had improved health if they had only accepted the teachings of Mrs. White.

"Finally, one can wonder how to make her teachings more widely known to benefit the overcrowded earth that seems inevitable tomorrow unless the present rate of increase of the world's population is decreased.

"In spite of the fact that the works of Mrs. White were written long before the advent of modern scientific nutrition, no better overall guide is available today." Clive McCay, Ph.D. Professor of Nutrition. 39

This is an introduction to some chapters later that are available online and the copyright has expired.

Thousands of years ago, the earliest Bible writer said, "The life of the flesh is in the blood" and man was to eat neither fat nor the blood of animals! Leviticus 3:17.

It has taken science more than 3,000 years to catch up, but close correlation of fat to coronary heart disease is now well established. If given a few more decades they might figure out that diseased animals (from the hormones and excreta fed to them) may be responsible for increases in cancer!

Nutrition is a factor in most disease. We are what we eat. Fads and foolish articles have confused millions for the sake of money. When you buy a car, you read the manual to learn what kind of fuel and oil you should use. The "Manufacturer's Manual" for man is the Bible.

In the very first chapter we learn that our original diet was composed of fruits, grains and nuts. After man sinned, herbs of the field, vegetables, were added. These foods, prepared in as simple and natural a manner as possible, free from oil or grease, are best for health.

1. Follow man's original diet as closely as possible.

2. Eat little of highly refined, fast or processed foods.

3. Learn to enjoy foods in their natural state with minimal cooking. Beans or grains should be well cooked.

4. Avoid salty or highly seasoned foods. They irritate the stomach and inflame the blood.

5. Avoid too many foods or combinations at one meal. Two or three are enough, four is plenty. Variety tends to provoke us to overeating with a result also of indigestion, sluggishness, or gas. Here an example:

For breakfast, have a generous serving of whole grain cereal and one or more slices of whole grain toast with a thin spread of nut butter or topped with sliced fruit or sauce like your cereal! Fresh fruit is better than juice; have all you wish! Avoid coffee, sugar or syrup, butter or margarine.

For dinner (mid-afternoon if possible as shown below), have generous servings of a starchy food (like potato, squash, rice or corn), and well-cooked beans or peas for protein plus something green (like spinach or kale) or yellow (carrots or squash) for vitamins. Fruit may be used if not having potatoes—it is better not to mix fruits and vegetables. Beans and peas are legumes, squash comes from a blossom and is the fruit of a vine, and rice or corn are grains, not vegetables!

6. Two meals a day is ideal for most people with the main meal at breakfast or early afternoon. This avoids the need of supper which is usually the most difficult to digest and the meal that tends to make us overweight. If a third meal is eaten, it should be light and several hours before retiring. (You don't drive your car all day on empty and then tank up after you get home.)

7. Have regular mealtimes, eat slowly, chew your food well. This helps prevent overeating and enables pleasant conversation. Avoid strenuous exercise right after eating.

8. A starch-based diet that is high in grains and complex carbohydrates is best.

Whole grain breads are easier to digest if toasted. Wheat, oats, brown rice, corn, millet, barley and rye are grains that may be prepared in many ways and they nicely balance the protein of beans or peas in the diet.

9. Fruits or vegetables are best fresh or frozen. Canned fruit should have the syrup poured off unless there is a food shortage; then it provides calories that are needed.

10. Because of the increase of disease in animals, dairy or poultry products are a risky type of food and cannot be recommended.

11. With machinery, a lean fuel is usually better than a rich mixture. The same is true for us. Avoid or eat rich foods sparingly. This includes nuts if you have angina or diabetes.

12. The above foods are high in vitamins, minerals, fiber and protective (anticancer) factors. Eat a wide variety of them with thanksgiving to the Creator and your health will be better!

Exercise

Every nerve and muscle of our being was made for action. Health cannot be maintained if we stay inactive. Exercise equalizes the circulation and enables necessary changes in the blood which must circulate freely to exchange oxygen and expel impurities.

Practical work is more beneficial than a gymnastic workout. Young men need vigorous exercise, as do students, who should balance their mental activity with physical work. Lack of exercise contributes to indigestion and insomnia, nervous, emotional and mental disorders. If space permitted, we could list at least 20 benefits of aerobic exercise!

1. Exercise daily in the open air. Dress for the cold in winter!

2. Equalize muscle and brain work as much as possible.

3. Walking is one of the best exercises. Be vigorous enough to promote some huffing and puffing. The disposition to avoid exercise is a sign that death is stalking you; shake it off!

4. Therapeutic exercise for angina means walking to the point of mild chest pain and then slowing, but continue walking in the presence of mild symptoms. This is a potent stimulant for arteries to open up and they will do so rapidly if on a low fat, cholesterol diet. This is contrasted with danger of running for a plane after a breakfast of bacon or sausage and eggs--and coffee (arrhythmia).

Water

1. Drink 6—8 glasses (8 oz) of pure water daily. One or two warm or hot glasses 20 minutes before breakfast is an excellent aid to bowel regularity. Add a squeeze of lemon if you wish.

2. Do not drink at mealtimes. It dilutes digestive juices and makes digestion more difficult.

3. Daily bath is best, but two—three times/week is minimum— use sponge bath if need be.

4. Tepid bath will help lower fever and give more water by mouth. Unless fever is 104, do not give Tylenol or Advil unless seizures have been a problem, which is more frequent in small dehydrated infants.

Sunlight

There are at least a dozen benefits from sunshine, the best known perhaps is Vitamin D, the sunshine vitamin which aids calcium metabolism, helping you absorb more from your food. Sunlight converts the cholesterol molecule to vitamin D, thus lowering cholesterol, and it also helps lowers blood pressure and blood sugar as a benefit to diabetics and hypertensives. It helps prevent infection, fight germs and aids hormonal balance.

1. Get as much sunshine as prudently possible. It is the polyunsaturated oils that have contributed to skin cancer. If you don't use much oil, moderate sun exposure won't hurt—it's been around for thousands of years!

2. Expose the rooms of the house to sunlight. It is great for mental attitude as well as health. Turn back the sheets, etc.

4. Plant some seeds that can give you food in return for the sunlight! Try alfalfa sprouts-—do it yourself!

Temperance

True temperance means to shun those things which are harmful, avoid extremes in anything, and be moderate in wholesome pleasures. Health is impossible without living under the control of enlightened reason. Sexual intemperance tends to paralyze the nerves and brain, causing loss of memory and life force.

The use of alcohol, tobacco or drugs, even drug "medication" will weaken the system. Human nature tends to be intemperate and we need God's help like in the 12 steps in Alcoholics Anonymous.

Air

Air is the most essential ingredient of life, yet millions get a marginal amount of air due to improper breathing. "In order to have good blood, we must breathe well. Full, deep inspirations of pure air, which fill the lungs with oxygen, purify the blood. They impart to it a bright color and send it, a life-giving current, to every part of the body.

A good respiration soothes the nerves; it stimulates the appetite and renders digestion more perfect; and it induces sound, refreshing sleep... (it) an insufficient supply of oxygen is received, the blood moves sluggishly.

The waste, poisonous matter, which should be thrown off in the exhalations from the lungs, is retained, and the blood becomes impure. Not only the lungs, but the stomach, liver, and brain are affected. The skin becomes sallow, digestion is retarded; the heart is depressed; the brain is clouded; the thoughts are confused; gloom settles upon the spirits; the whole system becomes depressed and inactive, and peculiarly susceptible to disease." *The Ministry of Healing*

1. In order to breathe well, you must have a correct posture in standing and sitting. God made man upright, and an erect bearing carries not only the grace and dignity of self-possession, but it promotes physical health and mental alertness. We should stand and walk tall because we were made in the image of God. Genesis 1:27.

2. Avoid tobacco in any form, and tight belts or garments that restrict deep respiration.

3. Develop the habit of deep breathing and always speak from the diaphragm using full inspirations.

4. Avoid overcrowded or poorly ventilated rooms. Get as much fresh air as possible. Many people could double the amount of good air they get by sleeping with a window open.

5. Do not overheat the house/apartment, as it removes the oxygen. Sixty-five to seventy degrees is the best temperature. You can dress warmer and still have better health and a clear mind.

6. Get some aerobic exercise (that makes you breathe heavily) daily. This tends to promote all of the remedies.

Rest

With hard work and exercise, there must be adequate rest. Rest is essential to restoration. Much of the benefit from medical care is really rest, absence of abuse, restoration of fluids, and time! During sleep, the body is repaired and the mind refreshed.

1. Have regular hours for sleep; going to bed early is best.

2. Deep breathing is an aid to sleeping better, but a large meal before retiring is not good.

3. "Count your blessings instead of sheep." A clear conscience, prayer, Bible study and trust in God are important aids to rest.

4. Avoid exciting programs or loud music. Excitement tends to derange the nervous system, like TV or fictional reading.

5. The Creator understood man's need to rest. So He made the night for this purpose. But if we cannot sleep or awaken early, reading the Bible or a good book can often relax the mind and enable one to go back to sleep.

6. Rest and wholesome diversion from weekly care and work may be found in the Sabbath that God made for our benefit. Mk 2:27.

Trust and Positive Attitudes

"Disease is sometimes produced, and is often greatly aggravated, by the imagination. Many are lifelong invalids who might be well if they only thought so...

Courage, hope, faith, sympathy, and love promote health and prolong life. A contented mind, a cheerful spirit, is health to the body and strength to the soul.

'A merry [rejoicing] heart does good like medicine.' Prov 17:22.

It has been estimated that 90% of disease has itS beginning in the mind, either by our choice of lifestyle or our habits of thought.

1. "What we don't use, we lose." We should use our minds to focus on tough problems or serious reading. Millions watch soap operas hoping to learn the meaning of life, and it soon becomes slippery. 'The Bible offers solid help that does not disappoint.

Novels or fiction are like junk food—it may taste good, but both mind and body are weakened by exciting trash. Like the stomach, the mind should have variation of food or it can become unbalanced. But much study promotes a weariness and our educational system focuses on memorization of facts to the detriment of mental health and real benefit.

2. The mind is more wonderful than the finest computer. It can discriminate between choices that are morally right or wrong. This power of choice is what makes our destiny as much higher than apes as the sun is higher than the earth.

God said, "Let us make man in our image, after our likeness." Genesis 1:26.

3. Realizing our potentially high destiny can give the most hopeful and spiritually exciting benefits to the mind. To realize that a loving Creator made us in His image and has provided the means whereby we may become sons and daughters by adoption into the heavenly family is the most fantastic truth that we can conceive.

In this case, "what the mind of man can conceive and believe, it can achieve!" So, let's "go for it!" The author has had 40 years experience in trusting the promises of Scripture, and I can tell you this; they work as well as any physics formula.

4. Let me clarify. God does not always give us just what we want when we want it.

For then He would be making us into overgrown babies, totally dependent upon our whim of "give me this" and "give me that." But in His great wisdom, He ordains what is best for us and will see us through any difficult situation, just in proportion to our trust and willingness to follow His way!

5. Like the computer we are programmed to do best when we look at things from a positive perspective. Dr. Selye, father of the modern stress theory, found that gratitude is one of the most healing of all emotions. And it is here where faith in Scripture can

46

be so meaningful, for one can express gratitude to the Creator for the high destiny that is ours and our belief that He is able to bring us to that expected end. Walking in the light that we have brings us to greater light.

6. Our feelings tend to follow our thoughts, like a caboose on a train. The caboose is not essential to the train— sometimes we see trains without one. In the same way, it is not necessary to feel great or high all the time.

If we focus on our feelings and fret because we are not feeling as high as we think we should, it is like focusing on the caboose and expecting it to run the train. We must focus on God's Word and His promises to us; our situation or perception of it will change.

7. "As a man thinks in his heart, so is he." Proverbs 23:7. If the thoughts run in a channel of fear, complaining, distrust, jealousy, or resentment, the body is toxic.

"An angry man is full of poison." Scripture says, "Whatsoever things are true, whatsoever things are honest, whatsoever things are just, whatsoever things are pure, whatsoever things are lovely, whatsoever things are of good report; if there be any virtue, and if there be any praise, think on these things." Philippians 4:8.

What has our attention has us. We become what we think about!

Summary

Health (one of our most important assets) costs us very little if we harmonize our lives with natural law. Doing so brings increased quality and quantity of life. This truth translates into the spiritual realm also. What we put into our minds can build us into better people, or corrupt us and lead to spiritual death.

Here's a link to a Natural Remedies Encyclopedia online so that you can get further help if you wish...

http://pathlights.com/nr_encyclopedia/index.htm

Diet and Health

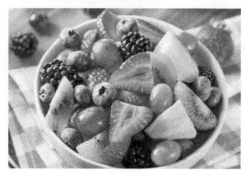

Our bodies are built up from the food we eat. There is a constant breaking down of the tissues of the body; every movement of every organ involves waste, and this waste is repaired from our food. Each organ of the body requires its share of nutrition. The brain must be supplied with its portion; the bones, muscles, and nerves demand theirs. It is a wonderful process that transforms the food into blood and uses this blood to build up the varied parts of the body; but this process is going on continually, supplying with life and strength each nerve, muscle, and tissue.

Selection of Food

Those foods should be chosen that best supply the elements needed for building up the body. In this choice, appetite is not a safe guide. Through wrong habits of eating, the appetite has become perverted. Often it demands food that impairs health and causes weakness instead of strength. We cannot safely be guided by the customs of society. The disease and suffering that everywhere prevail are largely due to popular errors in regard to diet.

In order to know what are the best foods, we must study God's original plan for man's diet. He who created man and who understands his needs appointed Adam his food. "Behold," He said, "I have given you every herb yielding seed, ... and every tree, in which is the fruit of a tree yielding seed; to you it shall be for food." Genesis 1:29, A.R.V. Upon leaving Eden to gain his livelihood by tilling the earth under the curse of sin, man received permission to eat also "the herb of the field." Genesis 3:18.

Grains, fruits, nuts, and vegetables constitute the diet chosen for us by our Creator. These foods, prepared in as simple and natural a manner as possible, are the most healthful and nourishing. They impart a strength, a power of endurance, and a vigor of intellect that are not afforded by a more complex and stimulating diet.

But not all foods wholesome in themselves are equally suited to our needs under all circumstances. Care should be taken in the selection of food. Our diet should be suited to the season, to the climate in which we live, and to the occupation we follow. Some foods that are adapted for use at one season or in one climate are not suited to another. So there are different foods best suited for persons in different occupations. Often food that can be used with benefit by those engaged in hard physical labor is unsuitable for persons of sedentary pursuits or intense mental application. God has given us an ample variety of healthful foods, and each person should choose from it the things that experience and sound judgment prove to be best suited to his own necessities.

Nature's abundant supply of fruits, nuts, and grains is ample, and year by year the products of all lands are more generally distributed to all, by the increased facilities for transportation. As a result many articles of food which a few years ago were regarded as expensive luxuries are now within the reach of all as foods for everyday use. This is especially the case with dried and canned fruits.

Nuts and nut foods are coming largely into use to take the place of flesh meats. With nuts may be combined grains, fruits, and some roots, to make foods that are healthful and nourishing. Care should be taken, however, not to use too large a proportion of nuts. Those who realize ill effects from the use of nut foods may find the difficulty removed by attending to this precaution. It

49

should be remembered, too, that some nuts are not so wholesome as others. Almonds are preferable to peanuts, but peanuts in limited quantities, used in connection with grains, are nourishing and digestible.

When properly prepared, olives, like nuts, supply the place of butter and flesh meats. The oil, as eaten in the olive, is far preferable to animal oil or fat. It serves as a laxative. Its use will be found beneficial to consumptives, and it is healing to an inflamed, irritated stomach.

Persons who have accustomed themselves to a rich, highly stimulating diet have an unnatural taste, and they cannot at once relish food that is plain and simple. It will take time for the taste to become natural and for the stomach to recover from the abuse it has suffered. But those who persevere in the use of wholesome food will, after a time, find it palatable. Its delicate and delicious flavors will be appreciated, and it will be eaten with greater enjoyment than can be derived from unwholesome dainties. And the stomach, in a healthy condition, neither fevered nor overtaxed, can readily perform its task.

In order to maintain health, a sufficient supply of good, nourishing food is needed.

If we plan wisely, that which is most conducive to health can be secured in almost every land. The various preparations of rice, wheat, corn, and oats are sent abroad everywhere, also beans, peas, and lentils. These, with native or imported fruits, and the variety of vegetables that grow in each locality, give an opportunity to select a dietary that is complete without the use of flesh meats.

Wherever fruit can be grown in abundance, a liberal supply should be prepared for winter, by canning or drying. Small fruits, such as currants, gooseberries, strawberries, raspberries, and blackberries, can be grown to advantage in many places where they are but little used and their cultivation is neglected.

For household canning, glass, rather than tin cans, should be used whenever possible. It is especially necessary that the fruit for canning should be in good condition. Use little sugar, and cook the fruit only long enough to ensure its preservation. Thus prepared, it is an excellent substitute for fresh fruit. Wherever dried fruits, such as raisins, prunes, apples, pears, peaches, and apricots are obtainable at moderate prices, it will be found that they can be used as staple articles of diet much more freely than is customary, with the best results to the health and vigor of all classes of workers.

There should not be a great variety at any one meal, for this encourages overeating and causes indigestion.

It is not well to eat fruit and vegetables at the same meal. If the digestion is feeble, the use of both will often cause distress and inability to put forth mental effort. It is better to have the fruit at one meal and the vegetables at another. {MH 299.7}

The meals should be varied. The same dishes, prepared in the same way, should not appear on the table meal after meal and day after day. The meals are eaten with greater relish, and the system is better nourished, when the food is varied.

Preparation of Food

It is wrong to eat merely to gratify the appetite, but no indifference should be manifested regarding the quality of the food or the manner of its preparation. If the food eaten is not relished, the body will not be so well nourished. The food should be carefully chosen and prepared with intelligence and skill.

For use in breadmaking, the superfine white flour is not the best. Its use is neither healthful nor economical. Fine-flour bread is lacking in nutritive elements to be found in bread made from the whole wheat. It is a frequent cause of constipation and other unhealthful conditions.

The use of soda or baking powder in bread-making is harmful and unnecessary. Soda causes inflammation of the stomach and often poisons the entire system. Many housewives think that they cannot make good bread without soda, but this is an error. If they would take the trouble to learn better methods, their bread would be more wholesome, and, to a natural taste, it would be more palatable. In the making of raised or yeast bread, milk should not be used in place of water. The use of milk is an additional expense, and it makes the bread much less wholesome. Milk bread does not keep sweet so long after baking as does that made with water, and it ferments more readily in the stomach.

Bread should be light and sweet. Not the least taint of sourness should be tolerated. The loaves should be small and so thoroughly baked that, so far as possible, the yeast germs shall be destroyed. When hot or new, raised bread of any kind is difficult of digestion. It should never appear on the table. This rule does not, however, apply to unleavened bread. Fresh rolls made of wheaten meal without yeast or leaven, and baked in a well-heated oven, are both wholesome and palatable.

Grains used for porridge or "mush" should have several hours' cooking. But soft or liquid foods are less wholesome than dry foods, which require thorough mastication. Zwieback, or twice-baked bread, is one of the most easily digested and most palatable of foods. Let ordinary raised bread be cut in slices and dried in a warm oven till the last trace of moisture disappears. Then let it be browned slightly all the way through. In a dry place this bread can be kept much longer than ordinary bread, and, if reheated before using, it will be as fresh as when new.

Far too much sugar is ordinarily used in food. Cakes, sweet puddings, pastries, jellies, jams, are active causes of indigestion. Especially harmful are the custards and puddings in which milk, eggs, and sugar are the chief ingredients. The free use of milk and sugar taken together should be avoided.

If milk is used, it should be thoroughly sterilized; with this precaution, there is less danger of contracting disease from its use. Butter is less harmful when eaten on cold bread than when used in cooking; but, as a rule, it is better to dispense with it altogether. Cheese is still more objectionable; it is wholly unfit for food.

Scanty, ill-cooked food depraves the blood by weakening the blood-making organs. It deranges the system and brings on disease, with its accompaniment of irritable nerves and bad tempers. The victims of poor cookery are numbered by thousands and tens of thousands. Over many graves might be written: "Died because of poor cooking;" "Died of an abused stomach."

It is a sacred duty for those who cook to learn how to prepare healthful food. Many souls are lost as the result of poor cookery. It takes thought and care to make good bread; but there is more religion in a loaf of good bread than many think. There are few really good cooks. Young women think that it is menial to cook and do other kinds of housework, and for this reason many girls who marry and have the care of families have little idea of the duties devolving upon a wife and mother.

Cooking is no mean science, and it is one of the most essential in practical life. It is a science that all women should learn, and it should be taught in a way to benefit the poorer classes. To make food appetizing and at the same time simple and nourishing, requires skill; but it can be done. Cooks should know how to prepare simple food in a simple and healthful manner, and so that it will be found more palatable, as well as more wholesome, because of its simplicity.

Every woman who is at the head of a family and yet does not understand the art of healthful cookery should determine to learn that which is so essential to the well-being of her household. In many places hygienic cooking schools afford opportunity for instruction in this line. She who has not the help of such facilities should put herself under the instruction of some good cook and persevere in her efforts for improvement until she is mistress of the culinary art.

Regularity in eating is of vital importance. There should be a specified time for each meal. At this time let everyone eat what the system requires and then take nothing more until the next meal. There are many who eat when the system needs no food, at irregular intervals, and between meals, because they have not sufficient strength of will to resist inclination. When traveling, some are constantly nibbling if anything eatable is within their reach. This is very injurious. If travelers would eat regularly of food that is simple and nutritious, they would not feel so great weariness nor suffer so much from sickness.

Another pernicious habit is that of eating just before bedtime. The regular meals may have been taken; but because there is a sense of faintness, more food is eaten. By indulgence this wrong practice becomes a habit and often so firmly fixed that it is thought impossible to sleep without food. As a result of eating late suppers, the digestive process is continued through the sleeping hours. But though the stomach works constantly, its work is not properly accomplished. The sleep is often disturbed with unpleasant dreams, and in the morning the person awakes unrefreshed and with little relish for breakfast. When we lie down to rest, the stomach should have its work all done, that it, as well as the other organs of the body, may enjoy rest. For persons of sedentary habits, late suppers are particularly harmful. With them the distur-bance created is often the beginning of disease that ends in death.

In many cases the faintness that leads to a desire for food is felt because the digestive organs have been too severely taxed during the day. After disposing of one meal, the digestive organs need rest. At least five or six hours should intervene between the meals, and most persons who give the plan a trial will find that two meals a day are better than three. {MH 304.1}

Wrong Conditions of Eating

Food should not be eaten very hot or very cold. If food is cold, the vital force of the stomach is drawn upon in order to warm it before digestion can take place. Cold drinks are injurious for the same reason; while the free use of hot drinks is debilitating. In fact, the more liquid there is taken with the meals, the more difficult it is for the food to digest; for the liquid must be absorbed before digestion can begin. Do not eat largely of salt, avoid the use of pickles and spiced foods, eat an abundance of fruit, and the irritation that calls for so much drink at mealtime will largely disappear.   54

Food should be eaten slowly and should be thoroughly masticated. This is necessary in order that the saliva may be properly mixed with the food and the digestive fluids be called into action.

Another serious evil is eating at improper times, as after violent or excessive exercise, when one is much exhausted or heated. Immediately after eating there is a strong draft upon the nervous energies; and when mind or body is heavily taxed just before or just after eating, digestion is hindered. When one is excited, anxious, or hurried, it is better not to eat until rest or relief is found.

The stomach is closely related to the brain; and when the stomach is diseased, the nerve power is called from the brain to the aid of the weakened digestive organs. When these demands are too frequent, the brain becomes congested. When the brain is constantly taxed, and there is lack of physical exercise, even plain food should be eaten sparingly. At mealtime cast off care and anxious thought; do not feel hurried, but eat slowly and with cheerfulness, with your heart filled with gratitude to God for all His blessings.

Many who discard flesh meats and other gross and injurious articles think that because their food is simple and wholesome they may indulge appetite without restraint, and they eat to excess, sometimes to gluttony. This is an error. The digestive organs should not be burdened with a quantity or quality of food which it will tax the system to appropriate.

Custom has decreed that the food shall be placed upon the table in courses. Not knowing what is coming next, one may eat a sufficiency of food which perhaps is not the best suited to him. When the last course is brought on, he often ventures to overstep the bounds, and take the tempting dessert, which, however, proves anything but good for him. If all the food intended for a meal is placed on the table at the beginning, one has opportunity to make the best choice. Sometimes the result of overeating is felt at once. In other cases there is no sensation of pain; but the digestive organs lose their vital force, and the foundation of physical strength is undermined.

The surplus food burdens the system and produces morbid, feverish conditions. It calls an undue amount of blood to the stomach, causing the limbs and extremities to chill quickly. It lays a heavy tax on the digestive organs, and when these organs have accomplished their task, there is a feeling of faintness or languor. Some who are continually overeating call this all-gone feeling hunger; but it is caused by the over-worked condition of the digestive organs. At times there is numbness of the brain, with disinclination to mental or physical effort.

These unpleasant symptoms are felt because nature has accomplished her work at an unnecessary outlay of vital force and is thoroughly exhausted. The stomach is saying, "Give me rest." But with many the faintness is interpreted as a demand for more food; so instead of giving the stomach rest, another burden is placed upon it. As a consequence the digestive organs are often worn out when they should be capable of doing good work.

We should not provide for the Sabbath a more liberal supply or a greater variety of food than for other days. Instead of this the food should be more simple, and less should be eaten in order that the mind may be clear and vigorous to comprehend spiritual things. A clogged stomach means a clogged brain. The most precious words may be heard and not appreciated because the mind is confused by an improper diet. By overeating on the Sabbath, many do more than they think to unfit themselves for receiving the benefit of its sacred opportunities.

Cooking on the Sabbath should be avoided; but it is not therefore necessary to eat cold food. In cold weather the food prepared the day before should be heated. And let the meals, however simple, be palatable and attractive. Especially in families where there are children, it is well, on the Sabbath, to provide something that will be regarded as a treat, something the family do not have every day.

Where wrong habits of diet have been indulged, there should be no delay in reform. When dyspepsia has resulted from abuse of the stomach, efforts should be made carefully to preserve the remaining strength of the vital forces by removing every overtaxing burden. The stomach may never entirely recover health after long abuse; but a proper course of diet will save further debility, and many will recover more or less fully. It is not easy to prescribe rules that will meet every case; but, with attention to right principles in eating, great reforms may be made, and the cook need not be continually toiling to tempt the appetite.

Abstemiousness in diet is rewarded with mental and moral vigor; it also aids in the control of the passions. Overeating is especially harmful to those who are sluggish in temperament; these should eat sparingly and take plenty of physical exercise. There are men and women of excellent natural ability who do not accomplish half what they might if they would exercise self-control in the denial of appetite.

Many writers and speakers fail here. After eating heartily, they give themselves to sedentary occupations, reading, study, or writing, allowing no time for physical exercise. As a consequence the free flow of thought and words is checked. They cannot write or speak with the force and intensity necessary in order to reach the heart; their efforts are tame and fruitless.

Those upon whom rest important responsibilities, those, above all, who are guardians of spiritual interests, should be men of keen feeling and quick perception. More than others, they need to be temperate in eating. Rich and luxurious food should have no place upon their tables.

Every day men in positions of trust have decisions to make upon which depend results of great importance. Often they have to think rapidly, and this can be done successfully by those only who practice strict temperance. The mind strengthens under the correct treatment of the physical and mental powers. If the strain is not too great, new vigor comes with every taxation. But often the work of those who have important plans to consider and important decisions to make is affected for evil by the results of improper diet. A disordered stomach produces a disordered, uncertain state of mind. Often it causes irritability, harshness, or injustice. Many a plan that would have been a blessing to the world has been set aside, many unjust, oppressive, even cruel measures have been carried, as the result of diseased conditions due to wrong habits of eating.

Here is a suggestion for all whose work is sedentary or chiefly mental; let those who have sufficient moral courage and self-control try it: At each meal take only two or three kinds of simple food, and eat no more than is required to satisfy hunger. Take active exercise every day, and see if you do not receive benefit.

Strong men who are engaged in active physical labor are not compelled to be as careful as to the quantity or quality of their food as are persons of sedentary habits; but even these would have better health if they would practice self-control in eating and drinking.

Some wish that an exact rule could be prescribed for their diet. They overeat, and then regret it, and so they keep thinking about what they eat and drink. This is not as it should be. One person cannot lay down an exact rule for another. Everyone should exercise reason and self-control, and should act from principle.

Our bodies are Christ's purchased possession, and we are not at liberty to do with them as we please. All who understand the laws of health should realize their obligation to obey these laws which God has established in their being. Obedience to the laws of health is to be made a matter of personal duty. We ourselves must suffer the results of violated law. We must individually answer to God for our habits and practices. Therefore the question with us is not, "What is the world's practice?" but, "How shall I as an individual treat the habitation that God has given me?"

Flesh as Food

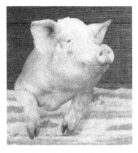

The diet appointed man in the beginning did not include animal food. Not till after the Flood, when every green thing on the earth had been destroyed, did man receive permission to eat flesh.

In choosing man's food in Eden, the Lord showed what was the best diet; in the choice made for Israel He taught the same lesson. He brought the Israelites out of Egypt and undertook their training, that they might be a people for His own possession. Through them He desired to bless and teach the world. He provided them with the food best adapted for this purpose, not flesh, but manna, "the bread of heaven." It was only because of their discontent and their murmuring for the fleshpots of Egypt that animal food was granted them, and this only for a short time. Its use brought disease and death to thousands. Yet the restriction to a nonflesh diet was never heartily accepted. It continued to be the cause of discontent and murmuring, open or secret, and it was not made permanent. Upon their settlement in Canaan, the Israelites were permitted the use of animal food, but under careful restrictions which tended to lessen the evil results. The use of swine's flesh was prohibited, as also of other animals and of birds and fish whose flesh was pronounced unclean. Of the meats permitted, the eating of the fat and the blood was strictly forbidden.

Only such animals could be used for food as were in good condition. No creature that was torn, that had died of itself, or from which the blood had not been carefully drained, could be used as food.

By departing from the plan divinely appointed for their diet, the Israelites suffered great loss. They desired a flesh diet, and they reaped its results. They did not reach God's ideal of character or fulfill His purpose. The Lord "gave them their request; but sent leanness into their soul." Psalm 106:15. They valued the earthly above the spiritual, and the sacred pre-eminence which was His purpose for them they did not attain.

Reasons for Discarding Flesh Foods

Those who eat flesh are but eating grains and vegetables at second hand; for the animal receives from these things the nutrition that produces growth. The life that was in the grains and vegetables passes into the eater. We receive it by eating the flesh of the animal. How much better to get it direct, by eating the food that God provided for our use!

Flesh was never the best food; but its use is now doubly objectionable, since disease in animals is so rapidly increasing. Those who use flesh foods little know what they are eating. Often if they could see the animals when living and know the quality of the meat they eat, they would turn from it with loathing. People are continually eating flesh that is filled with tuberculous and cancerous germs. Tuberculosis, cancer, and other fatal diseases are thus communicated.

The tissues of the swine swarm with parasites. Of the swine God said, "It is unclean unto you: ye shall not eat of their flesh, nor touch their dead carcass." Deuteronomy 14:8. This command was given because swine's flesh is unfit for food. Swine are scavengers, and this is the only use they were intended to serve. Never, under any circumstances, was their flesh to be eaten by human beings. It is impossible for the flesh of any living creature to be wholesome when filth is its natural element and when it feeds upon every detestable thing.

Often animals are taken to market and sold for food when they are so diseased that their owners fear to keep them longer. And some of the processes of fattening them for market produce disease. Shut away from the light and pure air, breathing the atmosphere of filthy stables, perhaps fattening on decaying food, the entire body soon becomes contaminated with foul matter.

Animals are often transported long distances and subjected to great suffering in reaching a market. Taken from the green pastures, and traveling for weary miles over the hot, dusty roads, or crowded into filthy cars, feverish and exhausted, often for many hours deprived of food and water, the poor creatures are driven to their death, that human beings may feast on the carcasses.

In many places fish become so contaminated by the filth on which they feed as to be a cause of disease. This is especially the case where the fish come in contact with the sewage of large cities. The fish that are fed on the contents of the drains may pass into distant waters and may be caught where the water is pure and fresh. Thus when used as food they bring disease and death on those who do not suspect the danger.

The effects of a flesh diet may not be immediately realized; but this is no evidence that it is not harmful. Few can be made to believe that it is the meat they have eaten which has poisoned their blood and caused their suffering. Many die of diseases wholly due to meat eating, while the real cause is not suspected by themselves or by others.

The moral evils of a flesh diet are not less marked than are the physical ills. Flesh food is injurious to health, and whatever affects the body has a corresponding effect on the mind and the soul. Think of the cruelty to animals that meat eating involves, and its effect on those who inflict and those who behold it. How it destroys the tenderness with which we should regard these creatures of God!

The intelligence displayed by many dumb animals approaches so closely to human intelligence that it is a mystery. The animals see and hear and love and fear and suffer. They use their organs far more faithfully than many human beings use theirs. They manifest sympathy and tenderness toward their companions in suffering. Many animals show an affection for those who have charge of them, far superior to the affection shown by some of the human race. They form attachments for man which are not broken without great suffering to them.

What man with a human heart, who has ever cared for domestic animals, could look into their eyes, so full of confidence and affection, and willingly give them over to the butcher's knife? How could he devour their flesh as a sweet morsel?

It is a mistake to suppose that muscular strength depends on the use of animal food. The needs of the system can be better supplied, and more vigorous health can be enjoyed, without its use. The grains, with fruits, nuts, and vegetables, contain all the nutritive properties necessary to make good blood. These elements are not so well or so fully supplied by a flesh diet. Had the use of flesh been essential to health and strength, animal food would have been included in the diet appointed man in the beginning.

When the use of flesh food is discontinued, there is often a sense of weakness, a lack of vigor. Many urge this as evidence that flesh food is essential; but it is because foods of this class are stimulating, because they fever the blood and excite the nerves, that they are so missed. Some will find it as difficult to leave off flesh eating as it is for the drunkard to give up his dram; but they will be the better for the change.

When flesh food is discarded, its place should be supplied with a variety of grains, nuts, vegetables, and fruits that will be both nourishing and appetizing. This is especially necessary in the case of those who are weak or who are taxed with continuous labor. In some countries where poverty abounds, flesh is the cheapest food. Under these circumstances the change will be made with greater difficulty; but it can be effected. We should, however, consider the situation of the people and the power of lifelong habit, and should be careful not to urge even right ideas unduly. None should be urged to make the change abruptly. The place of meat should be supplied with wholesome foods that are inexpensive. In this matter very much depends on the cook. With care and skill, dishes may be prepared that will be both nutritious and appetizing, and will, to a great degree, take the place of flesh food.

In all cases educate the conscience, enlist the will, supply good, wholesome food, and the change will be readily made, and the demand for flesh will soon cease.

Is it not time that all should aim to dispense with flesh foods? How can those who are seeking to become pure, refined, and holy, that they may have the companionship of heavenly angels, continue to use as food anything that has so harmful an effect on soul and body? How can they take the life of God's creatures that they may consume the flesh as a luxury? Let them, rather, return to the wholesome and delicious food given to man in the beginning, and themselves practice, and teach their children to practice, mercy toward the dumb creatures that God has made and has placed under our dominion.

Extremes in Diet

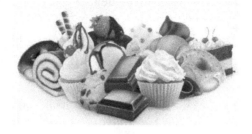

Not all who profess to believe in dietetic reform are really reformers. With many persons the reform consists merely in discarding certain unwholesome foods. They do not understand clearly the principles of health, and their tables, still loaded with harmful dainties, are far from being an example of Christian temperance and moderation.

Another class, in their desire to set a right example, go to the opposite extreme. Some are unable to obtain the most desirable foods, and, instead of using such things as would best supply the lack, they adopt an impoverished diet. Their food does not supply the elements needed to make good blood. Their health suffers, their usefulness is impaired, and their example tells against, rather than in favor of, reform in diet. Others think that since health requires a simple diet, there need be little care in the selection or the preparation of food. Some restrict themselves to a very meager diet, not having sufficient variety to supply the needs of the system, and they suffer in consequence.

Those who have but a partial understanding of the principles of reform are often the most rigid, not only in carrying out their views themselves, but in urging them on their families and their neighbors. The effect of their mistaken reforms, as seen in their own ill-health, and their efforts to force their views upon others, give many a false idea of dietetic reform, and lead them to reject it altogether.

Those who understand the laws of health and who are governed by principle, will shun the extremes, both of indulgence and of restriction. Their diet is chosen, not for the mere gratification of appetite, but for the up-building of the body. They seek to preserve every power in the best condition for highest service to God and man. The appetite is under the control of reason and conscience, and they are rewarded with health of body and mind. While they do not urge their views offensively upon others, their example is a testimony in favor of right principles. These persons have a wide influence for good.

There is real common sense in dietetic reform. The subject should be studied broadly and deeply, and no one should criticize others because their practice is not, in all things, in harmony with his own. It is impossible to make an unvarying rule to regulate everyone's habits, and no one should think himself a criterion for all. Not all can eat the same things. Foods that are palatable and wholesome to one person may be distasteful, and even harmful, to another. Some cannot use milk, while others thrive on it. Some persons cannot digest peas and beans; others find them wholesome. For some the coarser grain preparations are good food, while others cannot use them.

Those who live in new countries or in poverty-stricken districts, where fruits and nuts are scarce, should not be urged to exclude milk and eggs from their dietary. It is true that persons in full flesh and in whom the animal passions are strong need to avoid the use of stimulating foods. Especially in families of children who are given to sensual habits, eggs should not be used. But in the case of persons whose blood-making organs are feeble,—especially if other foods to supply the needed elements cannot be obtained,—milk and eggs should not be wholly discarded. Great care should be taken, however, to obtain milk from healthy cows, and eggs from healthy fowls, that are well fed and well cared for; and the eggs should be so cooked as to be most easily digested.

The diet reform should be progressive. As disease in animals increases, the use of milk and eggs will become more and more unsafe. An effort should be made to supply their place with other things that are healthful and inexpensive. The people everywhere should be taught how to cook without milk and eggs, so far as possible, and yet have their food wholesome and palatable.

The practice of eating but two meals a day is generally found a benefit to health; yet under some circumstances persons may require a third meal. This should, however, if taken at all, be very light, and of food most easily digested. "Crackers"—the English biscuit—or zwieback, and fruit, or cereal coffee, are the foods best suited for the evening meal.

Some are continually anxious lest their food, however simple and healthful, may hurt them. To these let me say, Do not think that your food will injure you; do not think about it at all. Eat according to your best judgment; and when you have asked the Lord to bless the food for the strengthening of your body, believe that He hears your prayer, and be at rest.

Because principle requires us to discard those things that irritate the stomach and impair health, we should remember that an impoverished diet produces poverty of the blood. Cases of disease most difficult to cure result from this cause. The system is not sufficiently nourished, and dyspepsia and general debility are the result. Those who use such a diet are not always compelled by poverty to do so, but they choose it through ignorance or negligence, or to carry out their erroneous ideas of reform.

God is not honored when the body is neglected or abused and is thus unfitted for His service. To care for the body by providing for it food that is relishable and strengthening is one of the first duties of the householder. It is far better to have less expensive clothing and furniture than to stint the supply of food.

Some householders stint the family table in order to provide expensive entertainment for visitors. This is unwise. In the entertainment of guests there should be greater simplicity. Let the needs of the family have first attention.

Unwise economy and artificial customs often prevent the exercise of hospitality where it is needed and would be a blessing.

The regular supply of food for our tables should be such that the unexpected guest can be made welcome without burdening the housewife to make extra preparation.

All should learn what to eat and how to cook it. Men, as well as women, need to understand the simple, healthful preparation of food. Their business often calls them where they cannot obtain wholesome food; then, if they have a knowledge of cookery, they can use it to good purpose.

Carefully consider your diet. Study from cause to effect. Cultivate self-control. Keep appetite under the control of reason. Never abuse the stomach by overeating, but do not deprive yourself of the wholesome, palatable food that health demands.

The narrow ideas of some would-be health reformers have been a great injury to the cause of hygiene. Hygienists should remember that dietetic reform will be judged, to a great degree, by the provision they make for their tables; and instead of taking a course that will bring discredit upon it, they should so exemplify its principles as to commend them to candid minds. There is a large class who will oppose any reform movement, however reasonable, if it places a restriction on the appetite. They consult taste instead of reason or the laws of health. By this class, all who leave the beaten track of custom and advocate reform will be accounted radical, no matter how consistent their course. That these persons may have no ground for criticism, hygienists should not try to see how different they can be from others, but should come as near to them as possible without sacrificing principle.

When those who advocate hygienic reform go to extremes, it is no wonder that many who regard these persons as representing health principles reject the reform altogether. These extremes frequently do more harm in a short time than could be undone by a lifetime of consistent living.

Hygienic reform is based upon principles that are broad and far-reaching, and we should not belittle it by narrow views and practices. But no one should permit opposition or ridicule, or a desire to please or influence others, to turn him from true principles, or cause him lightly to regard them.

Stimulants & Narcotics

Under the head of stimulants and narcotics is classed a great variety of articles that, altogether used as food or drink, irritate the stomach, poison the blood, and excite the nerves. Their use is a positive evil. Men seek the excitement of stimulants, because, for the time, the results are agreeable. But there is always a reaction. The use of unnatural stimulants always tends to excess, and it is an active agent in promoting physical degeneration and decay.

Condiments

In this fast age, the less exciting the food, the better. Condiments are injurious in their nature. Mustard, pepper, spices, pickles, and other things of a like character, irritate the stomach and make the blood feverish and impure. The inflamed condition of the drunkard's stomach is often pictured as illustrating the effect of alcoholic liquors. A similarly inflamed condition is produced by the use of irritating condiments. Soon ordinary food does not satisfy the appetite. The system feels a want, a craving, for something more stimulating.

Tea and Coffee

Tea acts as a stimulant and, to a certain extent, produces intoxication. The action of coffee and many other popular drinks is similar. The first effect is exhilarating. The nerves of the stomach are excited; these convey irritation to the brain, and this in turn is aroused to impart increased action to the heart and short-lived energy to the entire system. Fatigue is forgotten; the strength seems to be increased. The intellect is aroused, the imagination becomes more vivid.

Because of these results, many suppose that their tea or coffee is doing them great good. But this is a mistake. Tea and coffee do not nourish the system. Their effect is produced before there has been time for digestion and assimilation, and what seems to be strength is only nervous excitement. When the influence of the stimulant is gone, the unnatural force abates, and the result is a corresponding degree of languor and debility.

The continued use of these nerve irritants is followed by headache, wakefulness, palpitation of the heart, indigestion, trembling, and many other evils; for they wear away the life forces. Tired nerves need rest and quiet instead of stimulation and overwork. Nature needs time to recuperate her exhausted energies. When her forces are goaded on by the use of stimulants, more will be accomplished for a time; but, as the system becomes debilitated by their constant use, it gradually becomes more difficult to rouse the energies to the desired point. The demand for stimulants becomes more difficult to control, until the will is overborne and there seems to be no power to deny the unnatural craving. Stronger and still stronger stimulants are called for, until exhausted nature can no longer respond.

The Tobacco Habit

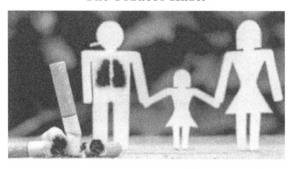

Tobacco is a slow, insidious, but most malignant poison. In whatever form it is used, it tells upon the constitution; it is all the more dangerous because its effects are slow and at first hardly perceptible. It excites and then paralyzes the nerves. It weakens and clouds the brain. Often it affects the nerves in a more powerful manner than does intoxicating drink. It is more subtle, and its effects are difficult to eradicate from the system. Its use excites a thirst for strong drink and in many cases lays the foundation for the liquor habit.

The use of tobacco is inconvenient, expensive, uncleanly, defiling to the user, and offensive to others. Its devotees are encountered everywhere. You rarely pass through a crowd but some smoker puffs his poisoned breath in your face. It is unpleasant and unhealthful to remain in a railway car or in a room where the atmosphere is laden with the fumes of liquor and tobacco. Though men persist in using these poisons themselves, what right have they to defile the air that others must breathe?

Among children and youth the use of tobacco is working untold harm. The unhealthful practices of past generations affect the children and youth of today. Mental inability, physical weakness, disordered nerves, and unnatural cravings are transmitted as a legacy from parents to children. And the same practices, continued by the children, are increasing and perpetuating the evil results. To this cause in no small degree is owing the physical, mental, and moral deterioration which is becoming such a cause of alarm.

Boys begin the use of tobacco at a very early age. The habit thus formed when body and mind are especially susceptible to its effects, undermines the physical strength, dwarfs the body, stupefies the mind, and corrupts the morals.

But what can be done to teach children and youth the evils of a practice of which parents, teachers, and ministers set them the example? Little boys, hardly emerged from babyhood, may be seen smoking their cigarettes. If one speaks to them about it, they say, "My father uses tobacco." They point to the minister or the Sunday-school superintendent and say, "Such a man smokes; what harm for me to do as he does?" Many workers in the temperance cause are addicted to the use of tobacco. What power can such persons have to stay the progress of intemperance?

I appeal to those who profess to believe and obey the word of God: Can you as Christians indulge a habit that is paralyzing your intellect and robbing you of power rightly to estimate eternal realities? Can you consent daily to rob God of service which is His due, and to rob your fellow men, both of service you might render and of the power of example?

Have you considered your responsibility as God's stewards, for the means in your hands? How much of the Lord's money do you spend for tobacco? Reckon up what you have thus spent during your lifetime. How does the amount consumed by this defiling lust compare with what you have given for the relief of the poor and the spread of the gospel?

No human being needs tobacco, but multitudes are perishing for want of the means that by its use is worse than wasted. Have you not been misappropriating the Lord's goods? Have you not been guilty of robbery toward God and your fellow men? "Know ye not that ... ye are not your own? For ye are bought with a price: therefore glorify God in your body, and in your spirit, which are God's." 1 Corinthians 6:19, 20.

71

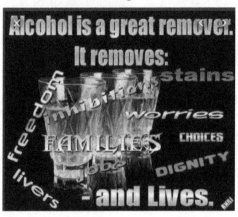

"Wine is a mocker, strong drink is raging:
And whosoever is deceived thereby is not wise."
"Who hath woe? who hath sorrow? who hath contentions?
who hath babbling? who hath wounds
without cause?
Who hath redness of eyes?
They that tarry long at the wine;
They that go to seek mixed wine.
Look not thou upon the wine when it is red,
When it giveth his color in the cup,
When it moveth itself aright.
At the last it biteth like a serpent,
And stingeth like an adder."

Proverbs 20:1; 23:29-32.

Never was traced by human hand a more vivid picture of the debasement and the slavery of the victim of intoxicating drink. Enthralled, degraded, even when awakened to a sense of his misery, he has no power to break from the snare; he "will seek it yet again." Verse 35.

No argument is needed to show the evil effects of intoxicants on the drunkard. The bleared, besotted wrecks of humanity—

souls for whom Christ died, and over whom angels weep—are everywhere. They are a blot on our boasted civilization. They are the shame and curse and peril of every land.

And who can picture the wretchedness, the agony, the despair, that are hidden in the drunkard's home? Think of the wife, often delicately reared, sensitive, cultured, and refined, linked to one whom drink transforms into a sot or a demon. Think of the children, robbed of home comforts, education, and training, living in terror of him who should be their pride and protection, thrust into the world, bearing the brand of shame, often with the hereditary curse of the drunkard's thirst.

Think of the frightful accidents that are every day occurring through the influence of drink. Some official on a railway train neglects to heed a signal or misinterprets an order. On goes the train; there is a collision, and many lives are lost. Or a steamer is run aground, and passengers and crew find a watery grave. When the matter is investigated, it is found that someone at an important post was under the influence of drink. To what extent can one indulge the liquor habit and be safely trusted with the lives of human beings? He can be trusted only as he totally abstains.

The Milder Intoxicants

Persons who have inherited an appetite for unnatural stimulants should by no means have wine, beer, or cider in their sight, or within their reach; for this keeps the temptation constantly before them. Regarding sweet cider as harmless, many have no scruples in purchasing it freely. But it remains sweet for a short time only; then fermentation begins. The sharp taste which it then acquires makes it all the more acceptable to many palates, and the user is loath to admit that it has become hard, or fermented.

There is danger to health in the use of even sweet cider as ordinarily produced. If people could see what the microscope reveals in regard to the cider they buy, few would be willing to drink it. Often those who manufacture cider for the market are not careful as to the condition of the fruit used, and the juice of wormy and decayed apples is expressed. Those who would not think of using the poisonous, rotten apples in any other way, will drink the cider made from them, and call it a luxury; but the microscope shows that even when fresh from the press, this pleasant beverage is wholly unfit for use. [When this statement was made in 1905, it was common practice to manufacture cider as here described by the author. Today, in places where the purity of foods is not controlled, apple cider may still be made the same way. But where cider is produced under sanitary conditions, using good, sound fruit, obviously the objections disappear.—Publishers.]

Intoxication is just as really produced by wine, beer, and cider as by stronger drinks. The use of these drinks awakens the taste for those that are stronger, and thus the liquor habit is established. Moderate drinking is the school in which men are educated for the drunkard's career. Yet so insidious is the work of these milder stimulants that the highway to drunkenness is entered before the victim suspects his danger.

Some who are never considered really drunk are always under the influence of mild intoxicants. They are feverish, unstable in mind, unbalanced. Imagining themselves secure, they go on and on, until every barrier is broken down, every principle sacrificed. The strongest resolutions are undermined, the highest considerations are not sufficient to keep the debased appetite under the control of reason.

The Bible nowhere sanctions the use of intoxicating wine. The wine that Christ made from water at the marriage feast of Cana was the pure juice of the grape. This is the "new wine ... found in the cluster," of which the Scripture says, "Destroy it not; for a blessing is in it." Isaiah 65:8.

It was Christ who, in the Old Testament, gave the warning to Israel, "Wine is a mocker, strong drink is raging: and whosoever is deceived thereby is not wise." Proverbs 20:1. He Himself provided no such beverage. Satan tempts men to indulgence that will becloud reason and benumb the spiritual perceptions, but

Christ teaches us to bring the lower nature into subjection. He never places before men that which would be a temptation. His whole life was an example of self-denial. It was to break the power of appetite that in the forty days' fast in the wilderness He suffered in our behalf the severest test that humanity could endure. It was Christ who directed that John the Baptist should drink neither wine nor strong drink. It was He who enjoined similar abstinence upon the wife of Manoah. Christ did not contradict His own teaching. The unfermented wine that He provided for the wedding guests was a wholesome and refreshing drink. This is the wine that was used by our Savior and His disciples in the first Communion. It is the wine that should always be used on the Communion table as a symbol of the Savior's blood. The sacramental service is designed to be soul-refreshing and life-giving. There is to be connected with it nothing that could minister to evil.

In the light of what the Scriptures, nature, and reason teach concerning the use of intoxicants, how can Christians engage in the raising of hops for beer making, or in the manufacture of wine or cider for the market? If they love their neighbor as themselves, how can they help to place in his way that which will be a snare?

Often intemperance begins in the home. By the use of rich, unhealthful food the digestive organs are weakened, and a desire is created for food that is still more stimulating. Thus the appetite is educated to crave continually something stronger. The demand for stimulants becomes more frequent and more difficult to resist. The system becomes more or less filled with poison, and the more debilitated it becomes, the greater is the desire for these things. One step in the wrong direction prepares the way for another. Many who would not be guilty of placing on their table wine or liquor of any kind will load their table with food which creates such a thirst for strong drink that to resist the temptation is almost impossible. Wrong habits of eating and drinking destroy the health and prepare the way for drunkenness.

There would soon be little necessity for temperance crusades if in the youth who form and fashion society, right principles in regard to temperance could be implanted. Let parents begin a crusade against intemperance at their own firesides, in the principles they teach their children to follow from infancy, and they may hope for success.

There is work for mothers in helping their children to form correct habits and pure tastes. Educate the appetite; teach the children to abhor stimulants. Bring your children up to have moral stamina to resist the evil that surrounds them. Teach them that they are not to be swayed by others, that they are not to yield to strong influences, but to influence others for good.

Great efforts are made to put down intemperance; but there is much effort that is not directed to the right point. The advocates of temperance reform should be awake to the evils resulting from the use of unwholesome food, condiments, tea, and coffee. We bid all temperance workers Godspeed; but we invite them to look more deeply into the cause of the evil they war against and to be sure that they are consistent in reform.

It must be kept before the people that the right balance of the mental and moral powers depends in a great degree on the right condition of the physical system. All narcotics and unnatural stimulants that enfeeble and degrade the physical nature tend to lower the tone of the intellect and morals. Intemperance lies at the foundation of the moral depravity of the world. By the indulgence of perverted appetite, man loses his power to resist temptation.

Temperance reformers have a work to do in educating the people in these lines. Teach them that health, character, and even life, are endangered by the use of stimulants, which excite the exhausted energies to unnatural, spasmodic action.

In relation to tea, coffee, tobacco, and alcoholic drinks, the only safe course is to touch not, taste not, handle not. The tendency of tea, coffee, and similar drinks is in the same direction as that of alcoholic liquor and tobacco, and in some cases the habit is as difficult to break as it is for the drunkard to give up intoxicants. Those who attempt to leave off these stimulants will for a time feel a loss and will suffer without them. But by persistence they will overcome the craving and cease to feel the lack. Nature may require a little time to recover from the abuse she has suffered; but give her a chance, and she will again rally and perform her work nobly and well.

Liquor Traffic and Prohibition

"Woe unto him that buildeth his house by unrighteousness, and his chambers by wrong; ... that saith, I will build me a wide house and large chambers, and cutteth him out windows; and it is ceiled with cedar, and painted with vermilion. Shalt thou reign, because thou closest thyself in cedar? ... Thine eyes and thine heart are not but for thy covetousness, and for to shed innocent blood, and for oppression, and for violence, to do it." Jeremiah 22:13-17.

The Work of the Liquor Seller

This scripture pictures the work of those who manufacture and who sell intoxicating liquor. Their business means robbery. For the money they receive, no equivalent is returned. Every dollar they add to their gains has brought a curse to the spender.

With a liberal hand, God has bestowed His blessings upon men. If His gifts were wisely used, how little the world would know of poverty or distress! It is the wickedness of men that turns His blessings into a curse. It is through the greed of gain and the lust of appetite that the grains and fruits given for our sustenance are converted into poisons that bring misery and ruin.

Every year millions upon millions of gallons of intoxicating liquors are consumed. Millions upon millions of dollars are spent in buying wretchedness, poverty, disease, degradation, lust, crime, and death. For the sake of gain, the liquor seller deals out to his victims that which corrupts and destroys mind and body. He entails on the drunkard's family poverty and wretchedness.

When his victim is dead, the rum seller's exactions do not cease. He robs the widow and brings children to beggary. He does not hesitate to take the very necessaries of life from the destitute family, to pay the drink bill of the husband and father. The cries of the suffering children, the tears of the agonized mother, serve

77

only to exasperate him. What is it to him if these suffering ones starve? What is it to him if they, too, are driven to degradation and ruin? He grows rich on the pittances of those whom he is leading to perdition.

Houses of prostitution, dens of vice, criminal courts, prisons, almshouses, insane asylums, hospitals, all are, to a great degree, filled as a result of the liquor seller's work. Like the mystic Babylon of the Apocalypse, he is dealing in "slaves, and souls of men." Behind the liquor seller stands the mighty destroyer of souls, and every art which earth or hell can devise is employed to draw human beings under his power. In the city and the country, on the railway trains, on the great steamers, in places of business, in the halls of pleasure, in the medical dispensary, even in the church, on the sacred Communion table, his traps are set. Nothing is left undone to create and to foster the desire for intoxicants. On almost every corner stands the public house, with its brilliant lights, its welcome and good cheer, inviting the working man, the wealthy idler, and the unsuspecting youth.

In private lunchrooms and fashionable resorts, ladies are supplied with popular drinks, under some pleasing name, that are really intoxicants. For the sick and the exhausted, there are the widely advertised bitters, consisting largely of alcohol.

To create the liquor appetite in little children, alcohol is introduced into confectionery. Such confectionery is sold in the shops. And by the gift of these candies the liquor seller entices children into his resorts.

Day by day, month by month, year by year, the work goes on. Fathers and husbands and brothers, the stay and hope and pride of the nation, are steadily passing into the liquor dealer's haunts, to be sent back wrecked and ruined.

More terrible still, the curse is striking the very heart of the home. More and more, women are forming the liquor habit. In many a household, little children, even in the innocence and helplessness of babyhood, are in daily peril through the neglect, the abuse, the vileness of drunken mothers. Sons and daughters are growing up under the shadow of this terrible evil. What outlook for their future but that they will sink even lower than their parents?

From so-called Christian lands the curse is carried to the regions of idolatry. The poor, ignorant savages are taught the use of liquor. Even among the heathen, men of intelligence recognize and protest against it as a deadly poison; but in vain have they sought to protect their lands from its ravages. By civilized peoples, tobacco, liquor, and opium are forced upon the heathen nations. The ungoverned passions of the savage, stimulated by drink, drag him down to degradation before unknown, and it becomes an almost hopeless undertaking to send missionaries to these lands.

Through their contact with peoples who should have given them a knowledge of God, the heathen are led into vices which are proving the destruction of whole tribes and races. And in the dark places of the earth the men of civilized nations are hated because of this.

The liquor interest is a power in the world. It has on its side the combined strength of money, habit, appetite. Its power is felt even in the church. Men whose money has been made, directly or indirectly, in the liquor traffic, are members of churches, "in good and regular standing." Churches that accept such members are virtually sustaining the liquor traffic. Too often the minister has not the courage to stand for the right. He does not declare to his people what God has said concerning the work of the liquor seller. To speak plainly would mean the offending of his congregation, the sacrifice of popularity and loss of salary.

The drunkard is capable of better things. He has been entrusted with talents with which to honor God and bless the world; but his fellow men have laid a snare for his soul and built themselves up by his degradation. They have lived in luxury while the poor victims whom they have robbed, lived in poverty and wretchedness. But God will require for this at the hand of him who has helped to speed the drunkard on to ruin.

The Home

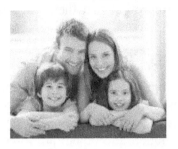

Ministry of the Home

The restoration and uplifting of humanity begins in the home. The work of parents underlies every other. Society is composed of families, and is what the heads of families make it. Out of the heart are "the issues of life" (Proverbs 4:23); and the heart of the community, of the church, and of the nation is the household. The well-being of society, the success of the church, the prosperity of the nation, depend upon home influences.

The importance and the opportunities of the home life are illustrated in the life of Jesus. He who came from heaven to be our example and teacher spent thirty years as a member of the household at Nazareth. Concerning these years the Bible record is very brief. No mighty miracles attracted the attention of the multitude. No eager throngs followed His steps or listened to His words. Yet during all these years He was fulfilling His divine mission. He lived as one of us, sharing the home life, submitting to its discipline, performing its duties, bearing its burdens. In the sheltering care of a humble home, participating in the experiences of our common lot, He "increased in wisdom and stature, and in favor with God and man." Luke 2:52.

During all these secluded years His life flowed out in currents of sympathy and helpfulness. His unselfishness and patient endurance, His courage and faithfulness, His resistance of temptation, His unfailing peace and quiet joyfulness, were a constant inspiration. He brought a pure, sweet atmosphere into the home, and His life was as leaven working amidst the elements of society. None said that He had wrought a miracle; yet virtue—the healing, life-giving power of love—went out from Him to the tempted, the sick, and the disheartened. In an unobtrusive way, from His very childhood, He ministered to others, and because of this, when He began His public ministry, many heard Him gladly.

The Savior's early years are more than an example to the youth. They are a lesson, and should be an encouragement, to every parent. The circle of family and neighborhood duties is the very first field of effort for those who would work for the uplifting of their fellow men. There is no more important field of effort than that committed to the founders and guardians of the home. No work entrusted to human beings involves greater or more far-reaching results than does the work of fathers and mothers.

It is by the youth and children of today that the future of society is to be determined, and what these youth and children shall be depends upon the home. To the lack of right home training may be traced the larger share of the disease and misery and crime that curse humanity. If the home life were pure and true, if the children who went forth from its care were prepared to meet life's responsibilities and dangers, what a change would be seen in the world!

Great efforts are put forth, time and money and labor almost without limit are expended, in enterprises and institutions for reforming the victims of evil habits. And even these efforts are inadequate to meet the great necessity. Yet how small is the result! How few are permanently reclaimed!

Multitudes long for a better life, but they lack courage and resolution to break away from the power of habit. They shrink from the effort and struggle and sacrifice demanded, and their lives are wrecked and ruined. Thus even men of the brightest minds, men of high aspirations and noble powers, otherwise fitted by nature and education to fill positions of trust and responsibility, are degraded and lost for this life and for the life to come.

For those who do reform, how bitter the struggle to regain their manhood! And all their life long, in a shattered constitution, a wavering will, impaired intellect, and weakened soul power, many reap the harvest of their evil sowing. How much more might be accomplished if the evil were dealt with at the beginning!

This work rests, in a great degree, with parents. In the efforts put forth to stay the progress of intemperance and of other evils that are eating like a cancer in the social body, if more attention were given to teaching parents how to form the habits and character of their children, a hundredfold more good would result. Habit, which is so terrible a force for evil, it is in their power to make a force for good. They have to do with the stream at its source, and it rests with them to direct it rightly.

Parents may lay for their children the foundation for a healthy, happy life. They may send them forth from their homes with moral stamina to resist temptation, and courage and strength to wrestle successfully with life's problems. They may inspire in them the purpose and develop the power to make their lives an honor to God and a blessing to the world. They may make straight paths for their feet, through sunshine and shadow, to the glorious heights above.

The mission of the home extends beyond its own members. The Christian home is to be an object lesson, illustrating the excellence of the true principles of life. Such an illustration will be a power for good in the world. Far more powerful than any sermon that can be preached is the influence of a true home upon human hearts and lives. As the youth go out from such a home, the lessons they have learned are imparted. Nobler principles of life are introduced into other households, and an uplifting influence works in the community.

There are many others to whom we might make our homes a blessing. Our social entertainments should not be governed by the dictates of worldly custom, but by the Spirit of Christ and the teaching of His word. The Israelites, in all their festivities, included the poor, the stranger, and the Levite, who was both the assistant of the priest in the sanctuary, and a religious teacher and missionary. These were regarded as the guests of the people, to share their hospitality on all occasions of social and religious rejoicing, and to be tenderly cared for in sickness or in need. It is such as these whom we should make welcome to our homes. How much such a welcome might do to cheer and encourage the missionary nurse or the teacher, the care-burdened, hard-working mother, or the feeble and aged, so often without a home, and struggling with poverty and many discouragements.

"When thou makest a dinner or a supper," Christ says, "call not thy friends, nor thy brethren, neither thy kinsmen, nor thy rich neighbors; lest they also bid thee again, and a recompense be made thee. But when thou makest a feast, call the poor, the maimed, the lame, the blind: and thou shalt be blessed; for they cannot recompense thee: for thou shalt be recompensed at the resurrection of the just." Luke 14:12-14.

These are guests whom it will lay on you no great burden to receive. You will not need to provide for them elaborate or expensive entertainment. You will need to make no effort at display. The warmth of a genial welcome, a place at your fireside, a seat at your home table, the privilege of sharing the blessing of the hour of prayer, would to many of these be like a glimpse of heaven.

Our sympathies are to overflow the boundaries of self and the enclosure of family walls. There are precious opportunities for those who will make their homes a blessing to others. Social influence is a wonderful power. We can use it if we will as a means of helping those about us.

Our homes should be a place of refuge for the tempted youth. Many there are who stand at the parting of the ways. Every influence, every impression, is determining the choice that shapes their destiny both here and hereafter. Evil invites them. Its resorts are made bright and attractive. They have a welcome for every comer. All about us are youth who have no home, and many whose homes have no helpful, uplifting power, and the youth drift into evil. They are going down to ruin within the shadow of our own doors. 83

These youth need a hand stretched out to them in sympathy. Kind words simply spoken, little attentions simply bestowed, will sweep away the clouds of temptation which gather over the soul. The true expression of heaven-born sympathy has power to open the door of hearts that need the fragrance of Christ-like words, and the simple, delicate touch of the spirit of Christ's love. If we would show an interest in the youth, invite them to our homes, and surround them with cheering, helpful influences, there are many who would gladly turn their steps into the upward path.

Life's Opportunities

Our time here is short. We can pass through this world but once; as we pass along, let us make the most of life. The work to which we are called does not require wealth or social position or great ability. It requires a kindly, self-sacrificing spirit and a steadfast purpose. A lamp, however small, if kept steadily burning, may be the means of lighting many other lamps. Our sphere of influence may seem narrow, our ability small, our opportunities few, our acquirements limited; yet wonderful possibilities are ours through a faithful use of the opportunities of our own homes. If we will open our hearts and homes to the divine principles of life we shall become channels for currents of life-giving power. From our homes will flow streams of healing, bringing life and beauty and fruitfulness where now are barrenness and dearth.

The Builders of the Home

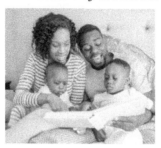

He who gave Eve to Adam as a helpmeet, performed His first miracle at a marriage festival. In the festal hall where friends and kindred rejoiced together, Christ began His public ministry. Thus He sanctioned marriage, recognizing it as an institution that He Himself had established. He ordained that men and women should be united in holy wedlock, to rear families whose members, crowned with honor, should be recognized as members of the family above.

Christ honored the marriage relation by making it also a symbol of the union between Him and His redeemed ones. He Himself is the Bridegroom; the bride is the church, of which, as His chosen one, He says, "Thou art all fair, My love; there is no spot in thee." Song of Solomon 4:7.

Christ "loved the church, and gave Himself for it; that He might sanctify and cleanse it; ... that it should be holy and without blemish." "So ought men to love their wives." Ephesians 5:25-28.

The family tie is the closest, the most tender and sacred, of any on earth. It was designed to be a blessing to mankind. And it is a blessing wherever the marriage covenant is entered into intelligently, in the fear of God, and with due consideration for its responsibilities.

Those who are contemplating marriage should consider what will be the character and influence of the home they are founding.

As they become parents, a sacred trust is committed to them. Upon them depends in a great measure the well-being of their children in this world, and their happiness in the world to come. To a great extent they determine both the physical and the moral stamp that the little ones receive. And upon the character of the home depends the condition of society; the weight of each family's influence will tell in the upward or the downward scale.

The choice of a life companion should be such as best to secure physical, mental, and spiritual well-being for parents and for their children—such as will enable both parents and children to bless their fellow men and to honor their Creator.

Before assuming the responsibilities involved in marriage, young men and young women should have such an experience in practical life as will prepare them for its duties and its burdens. Early marriages are not to be encouraged. A relation so important as marriage and so far-reaching in its results should not be entered upon hastily, without sufficient preparation, and before the mental and physical powers are well developed.

The parties may not have worldly wealth, but they should have the far greater blessing of health. And in most cases there should not be a great disparity in age. A neglect of this rule may result in seriously impairing the health of the younger. And often the children are robbed of physical and mental strength. They cannot receive from an aged parent the care and companionship which their young lives demand, and they may be deprived by death of the father or the mother at the very time when love and guidance are most needed.

It is only in Christ that a marriage alliance can be safely formed. Human love should draw its closest bonds from divine love. Only where Christ reigns can there be deep, true, unselfish affection.

Love is a precious gift, which we receive from Jesus. Pure and holy affection is not a feeling, but a principle. Those who are actuated by true love are neither unreasonable nor blind. Taught by the Holy Spirit, they love God supremely, and their neighbor as themselves.

Let those who are contemplating marriage weigh every sentiment and watch every development of character in the one with whom they think to unite their life destiny. Let every step toward a marriage alliance be characterized by modesty, simplicity, sincerity, and an earnest purpose to please and honor God. Marriage affects the afterlife both in this world and in the world to come. A Christian will make no plans that God cannot approve.

If you are blessed with God-fearing parents, seek counsel of them. Open to them your hopes and plans, learn the lessons which their life experiences have taught, and you will be saved many a heartache. Above all, make Christ your counselor. Study His word with prayer.

Under such guidance let a young woman accept as a life companion only one who possesses pure, manly traits of character, one who is diligent, aspiring, and honest, one who loves and fears God. Let a young man seek one to stand by his side who is fitted to bear her share of life's burdens, one whose influence will ennoble and refine him, and who will make him happy in her love.

"A prudent wife is from the Lord." "The heart of her husband doth safely trust in her.... She will do him good and not evil all the days of her life." "She openeth her mouth with wisdom; and in her tongue is the law of kindness. She looketh well to the ways of her household, and eateth not the bread of idleness. Her children arise up, and call her blessed; her husband also, and he praiseth her," saying, "Many daughters have done virtuously, but thou excellest them all." He who gains such a wife "findeth a good thing, and obtaineth favor of the Lord." Proverbs 19:14; 31:11, 12, 26-29; 18:22.

However carefully and wisely marriage may have been entered into, few couples are completely united when the marriage ceremony is performed. The real union of the two in wedlock is the work of the after years.

As life with its burden of perplexity and care meets the newly wedded pair, the romance with which imagination so often invests marriage disappears. Husband and wife learn each other's character as it was impossible to learn it in their previous association. This is a most critical period in their experience. The happiness and usefulness of their whole future life depend upon their taking a right course now. Often they discern in each other unsuspected weaknesses and defects; but the hearts that love has united will discern excellencies also heretofore unknown. Let all seek to discover the excellencies rather than the defects. Often it is our own attitude, the atmosphere that surrounds ourselves, which determines what will be revealed to us in another. There are many who regard the expression of love as a weakness, and they maintain a reserve that repels others. This spirit checks the current of sympathy. As the social and generous impulses are repressed, they wither, and the heart becomes desolate and cold. We should beware of this error. Love cannot long exist without expression. Let not the heart of one connected with you starve for the want of kindness and sympathy.

Though difficulties, perplexities, and discouragements may arise, let neither husband nor wife harbor the thought that their union is a mistake or a disappointment. Determine to be all that it is possible to be to each other. Continue the early attentions. In every way encourage each other in fighting the battles of life. Study to advance the happiness of each other. Let there be mutual love, mutual forbearance. Then marriage, instead of being the end of love, will be as it were the very beginning of love. The warmth of true friendship, the love that binds heart to heart, is a foretaste of the joys of heaven.

Around every family there is a sacred circle that should be kept unbroken. Within this circle no other person has a right to come. Let not the husband or the wife permit another to share the confidences that belong solely to themselves.

Let each give love rather than exact it. Cultivate that which is noblest in yourselves, and be quick to recognize the good qualities in each other. The consciousness of being appreciated is a wonderful stimulus and satisfaction. Sympathy and respect encourage the striving after excellence, and love itself increases as it stimulates to nobler aims.

Neither the husband nor the wife should merge his or her individuality in that of the other. Each has a personal relation to God. Of Him each is to ask, "What is right?" "What is wrong?" "How may I best fulfill life's purpose?" Let the wealth of your affection flow forth to Him who gave His life for you. Make Christ first and last and best in everything. As your love for Him becomes deeper and stronger, your love for each other will be purified and strengthened.

The spirit that Christ manifests toward us is the spirit that husband and wife are to manifest toward each other. "As Christ also hath loved us," "walk in love." "As the church is subject unto Christ, so let the wives be to their own husbands in everything. Husbands, love your wives, even as Christ also loved the church, and gave Himself for it." Ephesians 5:2, 24, 25.

Neither the husband nor the wife should attempt to exercise over the other an arbitrary control. Do not try to compel each other to yield to your wishes. You cannot do this and retain each other's love. Be kind, patient, and forbearing, considerate, and courteous. By the grace of God you can succeed in making each other happy, as in your marriage vow you promised to do.

Happiness in Unselfish Service

But remember that happiness will not be found in shutting yourselves up to yourselves, satisfied to pour out all your affection upon each other. Seize upon every opportunity for contributing to the happiness of those around you. Remember that true joy can be found only in unselfish service.

Forbearance and unselfishness mark the words and acts of all who live the new life in Christ. As you seek to live His life, striving to conquer self and selfishness and to minister to the needs of others, you will gain victory after victory. Thus your influence will bless the world.

Men and women can reach God's ideal for them if they will take Christ as their helper. What human wisdom cannot do, His grace will accomplish for those who give themselves to Him in loving trust. His providence can unite hearts in bonds that are of heavenly origin. Love will not be a mere exchange of soft and flattering words. The loom of heaven weaves with warp and woof finer, yet more firm, than can be woven by the looms of earth. The result is not a tissue fabric, but a texture that will bear wear and test and trial. Heart will be bound to heart in the golden bonds of a love that is enduring.

Better than gold is a peaceful home,
Where all the fireside charities come;
The shrine of love and the heaven of life,
Hallowed by mother, or sister, or wife.
However humble the home may be,
Or tried with sorrows by heaven's decree,
The blessings that never were bought or sold,
And center there, are better than gold. Anon.

Choice and Preparation of the Home

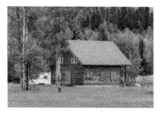

The gospel is a wonderful simplifier of life's problems. Its instruction, heeded, would make plain many a perplexity and save us from many an error. It teaches us to estimate things at their true value and to give the most effort to the things of greatest worth—the things that will endure. This lesson is needed by those upon whom rests the responsibility of selecting a home. They should not allow themselves to be diverted from the highest aim. Let them remember that the home on earth is to be a symbol of and a preparation for the home in heaven. Life is a training school, from which parents and children are to be graduated to the higher school in the mansions of God. As the location for a home is sought, let this purpose direct the choice. Be not controlled by the desire for wealth, the dictates of fashion, or the customs of society. Consider what will tend most to simplicity, purity, health, and real worth.

The world over, cities are becoming hotbeds of vice. On every hand are the sights and sounds of evil. Everywhere are enticements to sensuality and dissipation. The tide of corruption and crime is continually swelling. Every day brings the record of violence—robberies, murders, suicides, and crimes unnamable.

Life in the cities is false and artificial. The intense passion for money getting, the whirl of excitement and pleasure seeking, the thirst for display, the luxury and extravagance, all are forces that, with the great masses of mankind, are turning the mind from life's true purpose. They are opening the door to a thousand evils. Upon the youth they have almost irresistible power.

One of the most subtle and dangerous temptations that assail the children and youth in the cities is the love of pleasure.

91

Holidays are numerous; games and horse racing draw thousands, and the whirl of excitement and pleasure attracts them away from the sober duties of life. Money that should have been saved for better uses is frittered away for amusements.

Through the working of trusts, and the results of labor unions and strikes, the conditions of life in the city are constantly becoming more and more difficult. Serious troubles are before us; and for many families removal from the cities will become a necessity.

The physical surroundings in the cities are often a peril to health. The constant liability to contact with disease, the prevalence of foul air, impure water, impure food, the crowded, dark, unhealthful dwellings, are some of the evils to be met.

It was not God's purpose that people should be crowded into cities, huddled together in terraces and tenements. In the beginning He placed our first parents amidst the beautiful sights and sounds He desires us to rejoice in today. The more nearly we come into harmony with God's original plan, the more favorable will be our position to secure health of body, and mind, and soul.

An expensive dwelling, elaborate furnishings, display, luxury, and ease, do not furnish the conditions essential to a happy, useful life. Jesus came to this earth to accomplish the greatest work ever accomplished among men. He came as God's ambassador, to show us how to live so as to secure life's best results. What were the conditions chosen by the infinite Father for His Son? A secluded home in the Galilean hills; a household sustained by honest, self-respecting labor; a life of simplicity; daily conflict with difficulty and hardship; self-sacrifice, economy, and patient, gladsome service; the hour of study at His mother's side, with the open scroll of Scripture; the quiet of dawn or twilight in the green valley; the holy ministries of nature; the study of creation and providence; and the soul's communion with God—these were conditions and opportunities in Jesus' early life.

So with the great majority of the best and noblest men of all ages. Read the history of Abraham, Jacob, and Joseph, of Moses,

David, and Elisha. Study the lives of men of later times who have most worthily filled positions of trust and responsibility, the men whose influence has been most effective for the world's uplifting.

How many of these were reared in country homes. They knew little of luxury. They did not spend their youth in amusement. Many were forced to struggle with poverty and hardship. They early learned to work, and their active life in the open air gave vigor and elasticity to all their faculties. Forced to depend upon their own resources, they learned to combat difficulties and to surmount obstacles, and they gained courage and perseverance. They learned the lessons of self-reliance and self-control. Sheltered in a great degree from evil associations, they were satisfied with natural pleasures and wholesome companionships. They were simple in their tastes and temperate in their habits. They were governed by principle, and they grew up pure and strong and true. When called to their lifework, they brought to it physical and mental power, buoyancy of spirit, ability to plan and execute, and steadfastness in resisting evil, that made them a positive power for good in the world.

Better than any other inheritance of wealth you can give to your children will be the gift of a healthy body, a sound mind, and a noble character. Those who understand what constitutes life's true success will be wise betimes. They will keep in view life's best things in their choice of a home.

Instead of dwelling where only the works of men can be seen, where the sights and sounds frequently suggest thoughts of evil, where turmoil and confusion bring weariness and disquietude, go where you can look upon the works of God. Find rest of spirit in the beauty and quietude and peace of nature. Let the eye rest on the green fields, the groves, and the hills. Look up to the blue sky, unobscured by the city's dust and smoke, and breathe the invigorating air of heaven. Go where, apart from the distractions and dissipations of city life, you can give your children your companionship, where you can teach them to learn of God through His works, and train them for lives of usefulness.

Simplicity in Furnishing

Our artificial habits deprive us of many blessings and much enjoyment, and unfit us for living the most useful lives. Elaborate and expensive furnishings are a waste not only of money, but of that which is a thousand-fold more precious. They bring into the home a heavy burden of care and labor and perplexity.

What are the conditions in many homes, even where resources are limited and the work of the household rests chiefly on the mother? The best rooms are furnished in a style beyond the means of the occupants and unsuited to their convenience and enjoyment. There are expensive carpets, elaborately carved and daintily upholstered furniture, and delicate drapery. Tables, mantels, and every other available space are crowded with ornaments, and the walls are covered with pictures, until the sight becomes wearying. And what an amount of work is required to keep all these in order and free from dust! This work, and the other artificial habits of the family in its conformity to fashion, demand of the housewife unending toil.

In many a home the wife and mother has no time to read, to keep herself well informed, no time to be a companion to her husband, no time to keep in touch with the developing minds of her children. There is no time or place for the precious Savior to be a close, dear companion. Little by little she sinks into a mere household drudge, her strength and time and interest absorbed in the things that perish with the using. Too late she awakes to find herself almost a stranger in her own home. The precious opportunities once hers to influence her dear ones for the higher life, unimproved, have passed away forever.

Let the homemakers resolve to live on a wiser plan. Let it be your first aim to make a pleasant home. Be sure to provide the facilities that will lighten labor and promote health

and comfort. Plan for the entertainment of the guests whom Christ has bidden us welcome, and of whom He says, "Inasmuch as ye have done it unto one of the least of these My brethren, ye have done it unto Me." Matthew 25:40.

Furnish your home with things plain and simple, things that will bear handling, that can be easily kept clean, and that can be replaced without great expense. By exercising taste, you can make a very simple home attractive and inviting, if love and contentment are there.

God loves the beautiful. He has clothed the earth and the heavens with beauty, and with a Father's joy He watches the delight of His children in the things that He has made. He desires us to surround our homes with the beauty of natural things.

Nearly all dwellers in the country, however poor, could have about their homes a bit of grassy lawn, a few shade trees, flowering shrubbery, or fragrant blossoms. And far more than any artificial adorning will they minister to the happiness of the household. They will bring into the home life a softening, refining influence, strengthening the love of nature, and drawing the members of the household nearer to one another and nearer to God.

The Mother

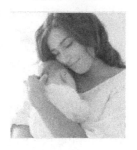

What the parents are, that, to a great extent, the children will be. The physical conditions of the parents, their dispositions and appetites, their mental and moral tendencies, are, to a greater or less degree, reproduced in their children.

The nobler the aims, the higher the mental and spiritual endowments, and the better developed the physical powers of the parents, the better will be the life equipment they give their children. In cultivating that which is best in themselves, parents are exerting an influence to mold society and to uplift future generations.

Fathers and mothers need to understand their responsibility. The world is full of snares for the feet of the young. Multitudes are attracted by a life of selfish and sensual pleasure. They cannot discern the hidden dangers or the fearful ending of the path that seems to them the way of happiness. Through the indulgence of appetite and passion, their energies are wasted, and millions are ruined for this world and for the world to come. Parents should remember that their children must encounter these temptations. Even before the birth of the child, the preparation should begin that will enable it to fight successfully the battle against evil.

Especially does responsibility rest upon the mother. She, by whose lifeblood the child is nourished and its physical frame built up, imparts to it also mental and spiritual influences that tend to the shaping of mind and character. It was Jochebed, the Hebrew mother, who, strong in faith, was "not afraid of the king's commandment" (Hebrews 11:23), of whom was born Moses, the deliverer of Israel. It was Hannah, the woman of prayer and self-sacrifice and heavenly inspiration, who gave birth to Samuel, the heaven-instructed child, the incorruptible judge, the founder of Israel's sacred schools. It was Elizabeth the kinswoman and kindred spirit of Mary of Nazareth, who was the mother of the Savior's herald.

Temperance and Self-Control

The carefulness with which the mother should guard her habits of life is taught in the Scriptures. When the Lord would raise up Samson as a deliverer for Israel, "the angel of Jehovah" appeared to the mother, with special instruction concerning her habits, and also for the treatment of her child. "Beware," he said, "and now drink no wine nor strong drink, neither eat any unclean thing." Judges 13:13, 7.

The effect of prenatal influences is by many parents looked upon as a matter of little moment; but heaven does not so regard it. The message sent by an angel of God, and twice given in the most solemn manner, shows it to be deserving of our most careful thought.

In the words spoken to the Hebrew mother, God speaks to all mothers in every age. "Let her beware," the angel said; "all that I commanded her let her observe." The well-being of the child will be affected by the habits of the mother. Her appetites and passions are to be controlled by principle. There is something for her to shun, something for her to work against, if she fulfills God's purpose for her in giving her a child. If before the birth of her child she is self-indulgent, if she is selfish, impatient, and exacting, these traits will be reflected in the disposition of the child. Thus many children have received as a birthright almost unconquerable tendencies to evil.

But if the mother unswervingly adheres to right principles, if she is temperate and self-denying, if she is kind, gentle, and unselfish, she may give her child these same precious traits of character. Very explicit was the command prohibiting the use of

97

wine by the mother. Every drop of strong drink taken by her to gratify appetite endangers the physical, mental, and moral health of her child, and is a direct sin against her Creator.

Many advisers urge that every wish of the mother should be gratified; that if she desires any article of food, however harmful, she should freely indulge her appetite. Such advice is false and mischievous. The mother's physical needs should in no case be neglected. Two lives are depending upon her, and her wishes should be tenderly regarded, her needs generously supplied. But at this time above all others she should avoid, in diet and in every other line, whatever would lessen physical or mental strength. By the command of God Himself she is placed under the most solemn obligation to exercise self-control.

Overwork

The strength of the mother should be tenderly cherished. Instead of spending her precious strength in exhausting labor, her care and burdens should be lessened. Often the husband and father is unacquainted with the physical laws which the well-being of his family requires him to understand. Absorbed in the struggle for a livelihood, or bent on acquiring wealth and pressed with cares and perplexities, he allows to rest upon the wife and mother burdens that overtax her strength at the most critical period and cause feebleness and disease.

Many a husband and father might learn a helpful lesson from the carefulness of the faithful shepherd. Jacob, when urged to undertake a rapid and difficult journey, made answer:

"The children are tender, and the flocks and herds with young are with me: and if men should overdrive them one day, all the flock will die.... I will lead on softly, according as the cattle that goeth before me and the children be able to endure." Genesis 33:13, 14.

In life's toilsome way let the husband and father "lead on softly," as the companion of his journey is able to endure. Amidst the world's eager rush for wealth and power, let him learn to stay his steps, to comfort and support the one who is called to walk by his side.

The mother should cultivate a cheerful, contented, happy disposition. Every effort in this direction will be abundantly repaid in both the physical well-being and the moral character of her children. A cheerful spirit will promote the happiness of her family and in a very great degree improve her own health.

Let the husband aid his wife by his sympathy and unfailing affection. If he wishes to keep her fresh and gladsome, so that she will be as sunshine in the home, let him help her bear her burdens. His kindness and loving courtesy will be to her a precious encouragement, and the happiness he imparts will bring joy and peace to his own heart.

The husband and father who is morose, selfish, and overbearing, is not only unhappy himself, but he casts gloom upon all the inmates of his home. He will reap the result in seeing his wife dispirited and sickly, and his children marred with his own unlovely temper.

If the mother is deprived of the care and comforts she should have, if she is allowed to exhaust her strength through overwork or through anxiety and gloom, her children will be robbed of the vital force and of the mental elasticity and cheerful buoyancy they should inherit. Far better will it be to make the mother's life bright and cheerful, to shield her from want, wearing labor, and depressing care, and let the children inherit good constitutions, so that they may battle their way through life with their own energetic strength.

Great is the honor and the responsibility placed upon fathers and mothers, in that they are to stand in the place of God to their children. Their character, their daily life, their methods of training, will interpret His words to the little ones. Their influence will win or repel the child's confidence in the Lord's assurances.

Happy are the parents whose lives are a true reflection of the divine, so that the promises and commands of God awaken in the child gratitude and reverence; the parents whose tenderness and justice and long-suffering interpret to the child the love and justice and long-suffering of God; and who, by teaching the child to love and trust and obey them, are teaching him to love and trust and obey his Father in heaven. Parents who impart to a child such a gift have endowed him with a treasure more precious than the wealth of all the ages—a treasure as enduring as eternity. {MH 375.3}

In the children committed to her care, every mother has a sacred charge from God. "Take this son, this daughter," He says; "train it for Me; give it a character polished after the similitude of a palace, that it may shine in the courts of the Lord forever."

The mother's work often seems to her an unimportant service. It is a work that is rarely appreciated. Others know little of her many cares and burdens. Her days are occupied with a round of little duties, all calling for patient effort, for self-control, for tact, wisdom, and self-sacrificing love; yet she cannot boast of what she has done as any great achievement. She has only kept things in the home running smoothly; often weary and perplexed, she has tried to speak kindly to the children, to keep them busy and happy, and to guide the little feet in the right path. She feels that she has accomplished nothing. But it is not so. Heavenly angels watch the care-worn mother, noting the burdens she carries day by day. Her name may not have been heard in the world, but it is written in the Lamb's book of life.

There is a God above, and the light and glory from His throne rests upon the faithful mother as she tries to educate her children to resist the influence of evil. No other work can equal hers in importance. She has not, like the artist, to paint a form of beauty upon canvas, nor, like the sculptor, to chisel it from marble. She has not, like the author, to embody a noble thought in words of power, nor, like the musician, to express a beautiful sentiment in melody. It is hers, with the help of God, to develop in a human soul the likeness of the divine.

The mother who appreciates this will regard her opportunities as priceless. Earnestly will she seek, in her own character and by her methods of training, to present before her children the highest

100

ideal. Earnestly, patiently, courageously, she will endeavor to improve her own abilities, that she may use aright the highest powers of the mind in the training of her children. Earnestly will she inquire at every step, "What hath God spoken?" Diligently she will study His word. She will keep her eyes fixed upon Christ, that her own daily experience, in the lowly round of care and duty, may be a true reflection of the one true Life.

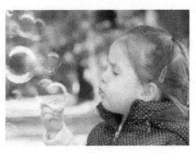

Not only the habits of the mother, but the training of the child were included in the angel's instruction to the Hebrew parents. It was not enough that Samson, the child who was to deliver Israel, should have a good legacy at his birth. This was to be followed by careful training. From infancy he was to be trained to habits of strict temperance.

Similar instruction was given in regard to John the Baptist. Before the birth of the child, the message sent from heaven to the father was: "Thou shalt have joy and gladness; and many shall rejoice at his birth. For he shall be great in the sight of the Lord, and he shall drink no wine nor strong drink; and he shall be filled with the Holy Spirit." Luke 1:14, 15, A.R.V.

On heaven's record of noble men the Saviour declared that there stood not one greater than John the Baptist. The work committed to him was one demanding not only physical energy and endurance, but the highest qualities of mind and soul. So important was right physical training as a preparation for this work that the highest angel in heaven was sent with a message of instruction to the parents of the child.

The directions given concerning the Hebrew children teach us that nothing which affects the child's physical well-being is to be neglected. Nothing is unimportant. Every influence that affects the health of the body has its bearing upon mind and character.

Too much importance cannot be placed upon the early training of children. The lessons learned, the habits formed, during the years of infancy and childhood, have more to do with the formation of the character and the direction of the life than have all the instruction and training of after years.

Parents need to consider this. They should understand the principles that underlie the care and training of children. They should be capable of rearing them in physical, mental, and moral health. Parents should study the laws of nature. They should become acquainted with the organism of the human body. They need to understand the functions of the various organs, and their relation and dependence. They should study the relation of the mental to the physical powers, and the conditions required for the healthy action of each. To assume the responsibilities of parenthood without such preparation is a sin.

Far too little thought is given to the causes underlying the mortality, the disease and degeneracy, that exist today even in the most civilized and favored lands. The human race is deteriorating.

Most of the evils that are bringing misery and ruin to the race might be prevented, and the power to deal with them rests to a great degree with parents. It is not a "mysterious providence" that removes the little children. God does not desire their death. He gives them to the parents to be trained for usefulness here, and for heaven hereafter. Did fathers and mothers do what they might to give their children a good inheritance, and then by right management endeavor to remedy any wrong conditions of their birth, what a change for the better the world might see!

The Care of Infants

The more quiet and simple the life of the child, the more favorable it will be to both physical and mental development. At all times the mother should endeavor to be quiet, calm, and self-possessed. Many infants are extremely susceptible to nervous excitement, and the mother's gentle, unhurried manner will have a soothing influence that will be of untold benefit to the child.

Babies require warmth, but a serious error is often committed in keeping them in overheated rooms, deprived to a great degree of fresh air. The practice of covering the infant's face while sleeping is harmful, since it prevents free respiration.

The baby should be kept free from every influence that would tend to weaken or to poison the system. The most scrupulous care should be taken to have everything about it sweet and clean. While it may be necessary to protect the little ones from sudden or too great changes of temperature, care should be taken, that, sleeping or waking, day or night, they breathe a pure, invigorating atmosphere.

In the preparation of the baby's wardrobe, convenience, comfort, and health should be sought before fashion or a desire to excite admiration. The mother should not spend time in embroidery and fancywork to make the little garments beautiful, thus taxing herself with unnecessary labor at the expense of her own health and the health of her child. She should not bend over sewing that severely taxes eyes and nerves, at a time when she needs much rest and pleasant exercise. She should realize her obligation to cherish her strength, that she may be able to meet the demands that will be made upon her.

If the dress of the child combines warmth, protection, and comfort, one of the chief causes of irritation and restlessness will be removed. The little one will have better health, and the mother will not find the care of the child so heavy a tax upon her strength and time.

Tight bands or waists hinder the action of the heart and lungs, and should be avoided. No part of the body should at any time be made uncomfortable by clothing that compresses any organ or restricts its freedom of movement. The clothing of all children should be loose enough to admit of the freest and fullest respiration, and so arranged that the shoulders will support its weight.

In some countries the custom of leaving bare the shoulders and limbs of little children still prevails. This custom cannot be too severely condemned. The limbs being remote from the center of circulation, demand greater protection than the other parts of the body. The arteries that convey the blood to the extremities are large, providing for a sufficient quantity of blood to afford warmth and nutrition. But when the limbs are left unprotected or are insufficiently clad, the arteries and veins become contracted, the sensitive portions of the body are chilled, and the circulation of the blood hindered.

In growing children all the forces of nature need every advantage to enable them to perfect the physical frame. If the limbs are insufficiently protected, children, and especially girls, cannot be out of doors unless the weather is mild. So they are kept in for fear of the cold. If children are well clothed, it will benefit them to exercise freely in the open air, summer or winter. Mothers who desire their boys and girls to possess the vigor of health should dress them properly and encourage them in all reasonable weather to be much in the open air. It may require effort to break away from the chains of custom, and dress and educate the children with reference to health; but the result will amply repay the effort.

The Child's Diet

The best food for the infant is the food that nature provides. Of this it should not be needlessly deprived. It is a heartless thing for a mother, for the sake of convenience or social enjoyment, to seek to free herself from the tender office of nursing her little one.

The mother who permits her child to be nourished by another should consider well what the result may be. To a greater or less degree the nurse imparts her own temper and temperament to the nursing child.

The importance of training children to right dietetic habits can hardly be overestimated. The little ones need to learn that they eat to live, not live to eat. The training should begin with the infant in its mother's arms. The child should be given food only at regular intervals, and less frequently as it grows older. It should not be given sweets, or the food of older persons, which it is unable to digest. Care and regularity in the feeding of infants will not only promote health, and thus tend to make them quiet and sweet-tempered, but will lay the foundation of habits that will be a blessing to them in after years.

As children emerge from babyhood, great care should still be taken in educating their tastes and appetite. Often they are permitted to eat what they choose and when they choose, without reference to health. The pains and money so often lavished upon unwholesome dainties lead the young to think that the highest object in life, and that which yields the greatest amount of happiness, is to be able to indulge the appetite. The result of this training is gluttony, then comes sickness, which is usually followed by dosing with poisonous drugs.

Parents should train the appetites of their children and should not permit the use of unwholesome foods. But in the effort to regulate the diet, we should be careful not to err in requiring children to eat that which is distasteful, or to eat more than is needed. Children have rights, they have preferences, and when these preferences are reasonable they should be respected.

Regularity in eating should be carefully observed. Nothing should be eaten between meals, no confectionery, nuts, fruits, or food of any kind. Irregularities in eating destroy the healthful tone of the digestive organs, to the detriment of health and cheerfulness. And when the children come to the table, they do not relish wholesome food; their appetites crave that which is hurtful for them.

Mothers who gratify the desires of their children at the expense of health and happy tempers, are sowing seeds of evil that will spring up and bear fruit. Self-indulgence grows with the growth of the little ones, and both mental and physical vigor are sacrificed. Mothers who do this work reap with bitterness the seed they have sown. They see their children grow up unfitted in mind and character to act a noble and useful part in society or in the home. The spiritual as well as the mental and physical powers suffer under the influence of unhealthful food. The conscience becomes stupefied, and the susceptibility to good impressions is impaired.

While the children should be taught to control the appetite and to eat with reference to health; let it be made plain that they are denying themselves only that which would do them harm. They give up hurtful things for something better. Let the table be made inviting and attractive, as it is supplied with the good things which God has so bountifully bestowed. Let mealtime be a cheerful, happy time. As we enjoy the gifts of God, let us respond by grateful praise to the Giver.

In many cases the sickness of children can be traced to errors in management. Irregularities in eating, insufficient clothing in the chilly evening, lack of vigorous exercise to keep the blood in healthy circulation, or lack of abundance of air for its purification, may be the cause of the trouble. Let the parents study to find the causes of the sickness, and then remedy the wrong conditions as soon as possible.

All parents have it in their power to learn much concerning the care and prevention, and even the treatment, of disease. Especially ought the mother to know what to do in common cases of illness in her family. She should know how to minister to her sick child. Her love and insight should fit her to perform services for it which could not so well be trusted to a stranger's hand.

The Study of Physiology

Parents should early seek to interest their children in the study of physiology and should teach them its simpler principles. Teach them how best to preserve the physical, mental, and spiritual powers, and how to use their gifts so that their lives may bring blessing to one another and honor to God. This knowledge is invaluable to the young. An education in the things that concern life and health is more important to them than a knowledge of many of the sciences taught in the schools.

Parents should live more for their children, and less for society. Study health subjects, and put your knowledge to a practical use. Teach your children to reason from cause to effect. Teach them that if they desire health and happiness, they must obey the laws of nature. Though you may not see so rapid improvement as you desire, be not discouraged, but patiently and perseveringly continue your work.

Teach your children from the cradle to practice self-denial and self-control. Teach them to enjoy the beauties of nature and in useful employments to exercise systematically all the powers of body and mind. Bring them up to have sound constitutions and good morals, to have sunny dispositions and sweet tempers. Impress upon their tender minds the truth that God does not design that we should live for present gratification merely, but for our ultimate good. Teach them that to yield to temptation is weak and wicked; to resist, noble and manly. These lessons will be as seed sown in good soil, and they will bear fruit that will make your hearts glad.

Above all things else, let parents surround their children with an atmosphere of cheerfulness, courtesy, and love. A home where love dwells, and where it is expressed in looks, in words, and in acts, is a place where angels delight to manifest their presence.

Parents, let the sunshine of love, cheerfulness, and happy contentment enter your own hearts, and let its sweet, cheering influence pervade your home. Manifest a kindly, forbearing spirit; and encourage the same in your children, cultivating all the graces that will brighten the home life. The atmosphere thus created will be to the children what air and sunshine are to the vegetable world, promoting health and vigor of mind and body.

Home Influences

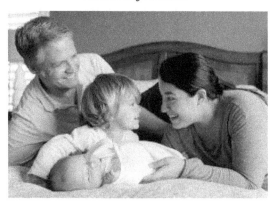

The home should be to the children the most attractive place in the world, and the mother's presence should be its greatest attraction. Children have sensitive, loving natures. They are easily pleased and easily made unhappy. By gentle discipline, in loving words and acts, mothers may bind their children to their hearts.

Young children love companionship and can seldom enjoy themselves alone. They yearn for sympathy and tenderness. That which they enjoy they think will please mother also, and it is natural for them to go to her with their little joys and sorrows. The mother should not wound their sensitive hearts by treating with indifference matters that, though trifling to her, are of great importance to them. Her sympathy and approval are precious. An approving glance, a word of encouragement or commendation, will be like sunshine in their hearts, often making the whole day happy.

Instead of sending her children from her, that she may not be annoyed by their noise or troubled by their little wants, let the mother plan amusement or light work to employ the active hands and minds.

By entering into their feelings and directing their amusements and employments, the mother will gain the confidence of her children, and she can the more effectually correct wrong habits, or check the manifestations of selfishness or passion. A word of caution or reproof spoken at the right time will be of great value. By patient, watchful love, she can turn the minds of the children in the right direction, cultivating in them beautiful and attractive traits of character.

Mothers should guard against training their children to be dependent and self-absorbed. Never lead them to think that they are the center, and that everything must revolve around them. Some parents give much time and attention to amusing their children, but children should be trained to amuse themselves, to exercise their own ingenuity and skill. Thus they will learn to be content with very simple pleasures. They should be taught to bear bravely their little disappointments and trials. Instead of calling attention to every trifling pain or hurt, divert their minds, teach them to pass lightly over little annoyances or discomforts. Study to suggest ways by which the children may learn to be thoughtful for others.

But let not the children be neglected. Burdened with many cares, mothers sometimes feel that they cannot take time patiently to instruct their little ones and give them love and sympathy. But they should remember that if the children do not find in their parents and in their home that which will satisfy their desire for sympathy and companionship, they will look to other sources, where both mind and character may be endangered.

For lack of time and thought, many a mother refuses her children some innocent pleasure, while busy fingers and weary eyes are diligently engaged on work designed only for adornment, something that, at best, will serve only to encourage vanity and extravagance in their young hearts. As the children approach manhood and womanhood, these lessons bear fruit in pride and moral worthlessness. The mother grieves over her children's faults, but does not realize that the harvest she is reaping is from seed which she herself planted.

Some mothers are not uniform in the treatment of their children. At times they indulge them to their injury, and again they refuse some innocent gratification that would make the childish heart very happy. In this they do not imitate Christ; He loved the children; He comprehended their feelings and sympathized with them in their pleasures and their trials.

The Father's Responsibility

The husband and father is the head of the household. The wife looks to him for love and sympathy, and for aid in the training of the children; and this is right. The children are his as well as hers, and he is equally interested in their welfare. The children look to their father for support and guidance; he needs to have a right conception of life and of the influences and associations that should surround his family; above all, he should be controlled by the love and fear of God and by the teaching of His word, that he may guide the feet of his children in the right way.

The father is the lawmaker of the household; and, like Abraham, he should make the law of God the rule of his home. God said of Abraham, "I know him, that he will command his children and his household." Genesis 18:19. There would be no sinful neglect to restrain evil, no weak, unwise, indulgent favoritism; no yielding of his conviction of duty to the claims of mistaken affection. Abraham would not only give right instruction, but he would maintain the authority of just and righteous laws. God has given rules for our guidance. Children should not be left to wander away from the safe path marked out in God's word, into ways leading to danger, which are open on every side. Kindly, but firmly, with persevering, prayerful effort, their wrong desires should be restrained, their inclinations denied.

The father should enforce in his family the sterner virtues— energy, integrity, honesty, patience, courage, diligence, and practical usefulness. And what he requires of his children he himself should practice, illustrating these virtues in his own manly bearing.

But, fathers, do not discourage your children. Combine affection with authority, kindness and sympathy with firm restraint. Give some of your leisure hours to your children;

become acquainted with them; associate with them in their work and in their sports, and win their confidence. Cultivate friendship with them, especially with your sons. In this way you will be a strong influence for good.

The father should do his part toward making home happy. Whatever his cares and business perplexities, they should not be permitted to overshadow his family; he should enter his home with smiles and pleasant words.

In a sense the father is the priest of the household, laying upon the family altar the morning and evening sacrifice. But the wife and children should unite in prayer and join in the song of praise. In the morning before he leaves home for his daily labor, let the father gather his children about him and, bowing before God, commit them to the care of the Father in heaven. When the cares of the day are past, let the family unite in offering grateful prayer and raising the song of praise, in acknowledgment of divine care during the day.

Fathers and mothers, however pressing your business, do not fail to gather your family around God's altar. Ask for the guardianship of holy angels in your home. Remember that your dear ones are exposed to temptations. Daily annoyances beset the path of young and old. Those who would live patient, loving, cheerful lives must pray. Only by receiving constant help from God can we gain the victory over self.

Home should be a place where cheerfulness, courtesy, and love abide; and where these graces dwell, there will abide happiness and peace. Troubles may invade, but these are the lot of humanity. Let patience, gratitude, and love keep sunshine in the heart, though the day may be ever so cloudy. In such homes angels of God abide.

Let the husband and wife study each other's happiness, never failing in the small courtesies and little kindly acts that cheer and brighten the life. Perfect confidence should exist between husband and wife. Together they should consider their responsibilities. Together they should work for the highest good

112

of their children. Never should they in the presence of the children criticize each other's plans or question each other's judgment. Let the wife be careful not to make the husband's work for the children more difficult. Let the husband hold up the hands of his wife, giving her wise counsel and loving encouragement.

No barrier of coldness and reserve should be allowed to arise between parents and children. Let parents become acquainted with their children, seeking to understand their tastes and dispositions, entering into their feelings, and drawing out what is in their hearts.

Parents, let your children see that you love them and will do all in your power to make them happy. If you do so, your necessary restrictions will have far greater weight in their young minds. Rule your children with tenderness and compassion, remembering that "their angels do always behold the face of My Father which is in heaven." Matthew 18:10. If you desire the angels to do for your children the work given them of God, co-operate with them by doing your part.

Brought up under the wise and loving guidance of a true home, children will have no desire to wander away in search of pleasure and companionship. Evil will not attract them. The spirit that prevails in the home will mold their characters; they will form habits and principles that will be a strong defense against temptation when they shall leave the home shelter and take their place in the world.

Children as well as parents have important duties in the home. They should be taught that they are a part of the home firm. They are fed and clothed and loved and cared for, and they should respond to these many mercies by bearing their share of the home burdens and bringing all the happiness possible into the family of which they are members.

Children are sometimes tempted to chafe under restraint; but in afterlife they will bless their parents for the faithful care and strict watchfulness that guarded and guided them in their years of inexperience.

113

True Education, a Missionary Training

True education is missionary training. Every son and daughter of God is called to be a missionary; we are called to the service of God and our fellow men; and to fit us for this service should be the object of our education.

Training for Service

This object should ever be kept in view by Christian parents and teachers. We know not in what line our children may serve. They may spend their lives within the circle of the home; they may engage in life's common vocations, or go as teachers of the gospel to heathen lands; but all are alike called to be missionaries for God, ministers of mercy to the world.

The children and youth, with their fresh talent, energy, and courage, their quick susceptibilities, are loved of God, and He desires to bring them into harmony with divine agencies. They are to obtain an education that will help them to stand by the side of Christ in unselfish service.

Of all His children to the close of time, no less than of the first disciples, Christ said, "As Thou hast sent Me into the world, even so have I also sent them into the world" (John 17:18), to be representatives of God, to reveal His Spirit, to manifest His character, to do His work.

Our children stand, as it were, at the parting of the ways. On every hand the world's enticements to self-seeking and self-indulgence call them away from the path cast up for the ransomed of the Lord. Whether their lives shall be a blessing or a curse depends upon the choice they make. Overflowing with energy, eager to test their untried capabilities, they must find some outlet for their super-abounding life. Active they will be for good or for evil.

God's word does not repress activity, but guides it aright. God does not bid the youth to be less aspiring. The elements of character that make a man truly successful and honored among men—the irrepressible desire for some greater good, the

114

indomitable will, the strenuous application, the untiring perseverance—are not to be discouraged. By the grace of God they are to be directed to the attainment of objects as much higher than mere selfish and worldly interests as the heavens are higher than the earth.

With us as parents and as Christians it rests to give our children right direction. They are to be carefully, wisely, tenderly guided into paths of Christ-like ministry. We are under sacred covenant with God to rear our children for His service. To surround them with such influences as shall lead them to choose a life of service, and to give them the training needed, is our first duty.

"God so loved, ... that He gave," "gave His only-begotten Son," that we should not perish, but have everlasting life. "Christ ... hath loved us, and hath given Himself for us." If we love we shall give. "Not to be ministered unto, but to minister" is the great lesson which we are to learn and to teach. John 3:16; Ephesians 5:2; Matthew 20:28.

Let the youth be impressed with the thought that they are not their own. They belong to Christ. They are the purchase of His blood, the claim of His love. They live because He keeps them by His power. Their time, their strength, their capabilities are His, to be developed, to be trained, to be used for Him.

Next to the angelic beings, the human family, formed in the image of God, are the noblest of His created works. God desires them to become all that He has made it possible for them to be, and to do their very best with the powers He has given them.

Life is mysterious and sacred. It is the manifestation of God Himself, the source of all life. Precious are its opportunities, and earnestly should they be improved. Once lost, they are gone forever.

Before us God places eternity, with its solemn realities, and gives us a grasp on immortal, imperishable themes. He presents valuable, ennobling truth, that we may advance in a safe and sure path, in pursuit of an object worthy of the earnest engagement of all our capabilities.   115

God looks into the tiny seed that He Himself has formed, and sees wrapped within it the beautiful flower, the shrub, or the lofty, wide-spreading tree. So does He see the possibilities in every human being. We are here for a purpose. God has given us His plan for our life, and He desires us to reach the highest standard of development.

He desires that we shall constantly be growing in holiness, in happiness, in usefulness. All have capabilities which they must be taught to regard as sacred endowments, to appreciate as the Lord's gifts, and rightly to employ. He desires the youth to cultivate every power of their being, and to bring every faculty into active exercise. He desires them to enjoy all that is useful and precious in this life, to be good and to do good, laying up a heavenly treasure for the future life.

It should be their ambition to excel in all things that are unselfish, high, and noble. Let them look to Christ as the pattern after which they are to be fashioned. The holy ambition that He revealed in His life they are to cherish—an ambition to make the world better for their having lived in it. This is the work to which they are called.

A Broad Foundation

The highest of all sciences is the science of soul saving. The greatest work to which human beings can aspire is the work of winning men from sin to holiness. For the accomplishment of this work, a broad foundation must be laid. A comprehensive education is needed—an education that will demand from parents and teachers such thought and effort as mere instruction in the sciences does not require. Something more is called for than the culture of the intellect. Education is not complete unless the body, the mind, and the heart are equally educated. The character must receive proper discipline for its fullest and highest development. All the faculties of mind and body are to be developed and rightly trained. It is a duty to cultivate and to exercise every power that will render us more efficient workers for God.

116

True education includes the whole being. It teaches the right use of one's self. It enables us to make the best use of brain, bone, and muscle, of body, mind, and heart. The faculties of the mind, as the higher powers, are to rule the kingdom of the body. The natural appetites and passions are to be brought under the control of the conscience and the spiritual affections. Christ stands at the head of humanity, and it is His purpose to lead us, in His service, into high and holy paths of purity. By the wondrous working of His grace, we are to be made complete in Him.

Jesus secured His education in the home. His mother was His first human teacher. From her lips, and from the scrolls of the prophets, He learned of heavenly things. He lived in a peasant's home and faithfully and cheerfully acted His part in bearing the household burdens. He who had been the commander of heaven was a willing servant, a loving, obedient son. He learned a trade and with His own hands worked in the carpenter's shop with Joseph. In the garb of a common laborer He walked the streets of the little town, going to and returning from His humble work.

With the people of that age the value of things was estimated by outward show. As religion had declined in power, it had increased in pomp. The educators of the time sought to command respect by display and ostentation. To all this the life of Jesus presented a marked contrast. His life demonstrated the worthlessness of those things that men regarded as life's great essentials. The schools of His time, with their magnifying of things small and their belittling of things great, He did not seek. His education was gained from Heaven- appointed sources, from useful work, from the study of the Scriptures, from nature, and from the experiences of life—God's lesson books, full of instruction to all who bring to them the willing hand, the seeing eye, and the understanding heart.

"The Child grew, and waxed strong in spirit, filled with wisdom: and the grace of God was upon Him." Luke 2:40.

Thus prepared, He went forth to His mission, in every moment of His contact with men exerting upon them an influence to bless, a power to transform, such as the world had never witnessed.

The home is the child's first school, and it is here that the foundation should be laid for a life of service. Its principles are to be taught not merely in theory. They are to shape the whole life training.

Very early the lesson of helpfulness should be taught the child. As soon as strength and reasoning power are sufficiently developed, he should be given duties to perform in the home. He should be encouraged in trying to help father and mother, encouraged to deny and to control himself, to put other's happiness and convenience before his own, to watch for opportunities to cheer and assist brothers and sisters and playmates, and to show kindness to the aged, the sick, and the unfortunate. The more fully the spirit of true ministry pervades the home, the more fully it will be developed in the lives of the children. They will learn to find joy in service and sacrifice for the good of others.

The Work of the School

The home training should be supplemented by the work of the school. The development of the whole being, physical, mental, and spiritual, and the teaching of service and sacrifice, should be kept constantly in view.

Above any other agency, service for Christ's sake in the little things of everyday experience has power to mold the character and to direct the life into lines of unselfish ministry. To awaken this spirit, to encourage and rightly to direct it, is the parents' and the teacher's work. No more important work could be committed to them. The spirit of ministry is the spirit of heaven, and with every effort to develop and encourage it angels will co-operate.

Such an education must be based upon the word of God. Here only are its principles given in their fullness. The Bible should be made the foundation of study and of teaching. The essential knowledge is a knowledge of God and of Christ whom He sent.

Every child and every youth should have a knowledge of himself. He should understand the physical habitation that God has given him, and the laws by which it is kept in health. All should be thoroughly grounded in the common branches of education. And they should have industrial training that will make them men and women of practical ability, fitted for the duties of everyday life. To this should be added training and practical experience in various lines of missionary effort.

Learning by Imparting

Let the youth advance as fast and as far as they can in the acquisition of knowledge. Let their field of study be as broad as their powers can compass. And, as they learn, let them impart their knowledge. It is thus that their minds will acquire discipline and power. It is the use they make of knowledge that determines the value of their education. To spend a long time in study, with no effort to impart what is gained, often proves a hindrance rather than a help to real development. In both the home and the school it should be the student's effort to learn how to study and how to impart the knowledge gained. Whatever his calling, he is to be both a learner and a teacher as long as life shall last. Thus he may advance continually, making God his trust, clinging to Him who is infinite in wisdom, who can reveal the secrets hidden for ages, who can solve the most difficult problems for minds that believe in Him.

God's word places great stress upon the influence of association, even upon men and women. How much greater is its power on the developing mind and character of children and youth. The company they keep, the principles they adopt, the habits they form, will decide the question of their usefulness here and of their future, eternal interest.

It is a terrible fact, and one that should make the hearts of parents tremble, that in so many schools and colleges to which the youth are sent for mental culture and discipline, influences prevail which misshape the character, divert the mind from life's true aims, and debase the morals. Through contact with the irreligious, the pleasure loving, and the corrupt, many, many

119

youth lose the simplicity and purity, the faith in God, and the spirit of self-sacrifice that Christian fathers and mothers have cherished and guarded by careful instruction and earnest prayer.

Many who enter school with the purpose of fitting themselves for some line of unselfish ministry become absorbed in secular studies. An ambition is aroused to win distinction in scholarship and to gain position and honor in the world. The purpose for which they entered school is lost sight of, and the life is given up to selfish and worldly pursuits. And often habits are formed that ruin the life both for this world and for the world to come.

As a rule, men and women who have broad ideas, unselfish purposes, noble aspirations, are those in whom these characteristics were developed by their associations in early years. In all His dealings with Israel, God urged upon them the importance of guarding the associations of their children. All the arrangements of civil, religious, and social life were made with a view to preserving the children from harmful companionship and making them, from their earliest years, familiar with the precepts and principles of the law of God. The object lesson given at the birth of the nation was of a nature deeply to impress all hearts. Before the last terrible judgment came upon the Egyptians in the death of the first-born, God commanded His people to gather their children into their own homes. The doorpost of every house was marked with blood, and within the protection assured by this token all were to abide. So today parents who love and fear God are to keep their children under "the bond of the covenant" — within the protection of those sacred influences made possible through Christ's redeeming blood. "Be not conformed to this world," God bids us; "but be ye transformed by the renewing of your mind." Romans 12:2.

"Be ye not unequally yoked together with unbelievers: for what fellowship hath righteousness with unrighteousness? and what communion hath light with darkness? ... and what agreement hath the temple of God with idols? for ye are the temple of the living God; as God hath said, I will dwell in them, and walk in them; and I will be their God, and they shall be My people. Wherefore

"Come out from among them, and be ye separate, ...
And touch not the unclean; And I will receive you, and
will be a Father unto you, And ye shall be My children.
Saith the Lord Almighty." 2 Corinthians 6:14-18.

Note: We are coming to a time when judgment may fall on the US as it did on Egypt when those who wanted to be God's people were separated in the Exodus. The Bible suggests a parallel event for end-times in 1Corinthians 10:1,11.

Summary: As a physician who taught Health Science at Loma Linda University, I see that most people should appreciate the previous information: Health comes from obedience to physical laws; And Happiness will result from Health and the obedience to moral laws.

There's one more topic related to happiness before we look at some Bible information that's important. It's about success...

Success!

Success is the progressive realization of a worthy goal. Most people equate money with success, but it doesn't have to be that way. Anyone who wants to be a good spouse or parent, or a teacher, for example, can be a success without getting rich.

Money in itself is a deceptive source of happiness--it's good for happiness only if used wisely. Ron Blue, a CPA with very wealthy clients, said they all wanted to know how much more they needed to be "secure." That says they misunderstand life.

A closely related truth is that we become what we think about and we need a goal to focus on. The long term goal can be broken up into short term goals like high school and college.

Using our time well each day helps us move toward our goal. If we waste our time, we are wasting our lives. "So teach us to number our days, that we may apply our hearts unto wisdom." Psalm 90:12. This brings us to the final section that is also related to happiness and destiny...

Not Left Behind!

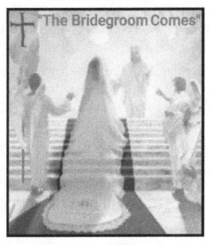

Dedication

This short book is dedicated to millions of Christians who don't want to be left behind. Millions of Catholics love Christ and are doing the best they know. Millions of Evangelicals may also wonder where this world is headed.

Left behind implies loneliness, and millions of Christians are lonely. They may be single folks who haven't married, or may be like me after my wife died, wanting to get married again.

Another deserving group to not leave behind are patriots who hate what's happening to the US and want to take the country back to what it was.

**The above groups and more are addressed in the Appendix.

"Christian" means those who live in pursuit of Christ who said He was the Truth, John 14:6. If you want to know the truth of the times, this book is for you and you will be blessed as you consider our journey together.

Contents

The following six parables have "9/11" timing, Numbers 9:10,11.

Introduction to Wow, How, When & Why!

#1. Why is easy. Just like parents love their kids and are excited to see in them a resemblance to themselves, the Bible says we are made in God's image. He loves us and has a wonderful plan for us, in spite of big mistakes made long ago...

#2. The Wow is Amos 3:7--"Surely the Lord God will do nothing but He reveals His secret to His servants, the prophets." The next verse is what He wants to reveal--it's about a lion's roar.

Christ is the Lion of Judah in Revelation 5:5. "The Lord shall roar...the earth shall shake." Joel 3:16. It's about an earthquake that will soon initiate the end-time "day of the Lord" as seen when God will "shake terribly the earth," Isaiah 2:12,21. Also Joel 2:10,11; Thessalonians 5:2,3.

#3. The How is about God's ability to foresee the repeat of history. He "declares the end from the beginning," (Isaiah 46:10) and the book of Genesis has more than "as the days of Noah."

"What is to come has been already, and God summons each event back in its turn," Ecclesiastes 3:15, New English Bible.

We focus on coming events in their order or in a logical sequence #4. The "when" is included because of God's ability to appoint times in the Bible that the Apostle Paul said "are shadows of things to come," Colossians 2:17.

An example is Passover, first seen in Exodus 12, when Israel was liberated from bondage and they went to the Promised Land, Passover began on the eve of the 15th day of Abib (the first spring month beginning with the new moon after the equinox). Israelites killed and ate a lamb on that night.

But nearly 1500 years later, a Hebrew prophet announced "the Lamb of God that takes away the sin of the world," John 1:29. Three and a half years later, Christ was slain as the Passover lamb to liberate a lost world from the bondage of sin.

A further example of God's appointed times is how 9/11 clues in Christ's last six parables signal when and how end-times begin.

126

It's God's 9/11 in Numbers 9:10,11 that are provisions for Passover as a time of judgment, but a month later, "as the days of Noah," Matthew 24:37. More on this later.

Christ said, "Many will say to me in that day, Lord, Lord, have we not...done many wonderful works? And then will I say to them, I never knew you." Matthew 7:22,23.

How could that be? Will Christ have amnesia? How could He not know, or what did He mean?

The key to understanding is in the Greek word, *ginosko*. It means knowing as in marriage or a covenant like Israel made with God after the Exodus and He later said, "I am married to you." Jeremiah 3:14.

This is a huge clue that we miss if we think the wedding parables are about a sudden trip to heaven. If that's where the marriage is, will He tell some in heaven, "I never knew you" when they knock on the door? Matthew 25:11,12.

The apostle Paul offers insight by including the Exodus in "all those things happened to them for [our] examples...ends of the world." 1Corinthians 10:*1*,11

History doesn't "repeat," but it rhymes with similar events as God "declares the end from the beginning." Isaiah 46:10.

The wedding parables are misunderstood as a sudden rapture before trouble comes. We will see later that it comes "at the last trumpet" in 1Corinthians 15:51,52. Revelation 8:5,6 shows seven trumpets come after a huge earthquake.

We need to see the wedding from a biblical view as when God "executed judgment" on Egypt and took Israel to a covenant by which they became His kingdom and Bride, Jeremiah 3:14.

Egypt killed babies but the US has aborted 60 million and enslaved most of its population in alcohol, tobacco, drugs and negative lifestyles.

Egypt also had seven good years followed by seven years of famine. America is seeing the good years with a good economy under Trump, but they will be followed by seven bad years.

President Trump may also be seen in Daniel 8. Most historians say that vision was fulfilled by Alexander the Great in the Battle of Arbela as he conquered the Medes and Persians in 331 BC.

But Gabriel told Daniel, "the vision is <u>at the time of the end</u>," Daniel 8:17,20. The Medes and Persians are Iraq and Iran--'time of the end.'

If you aren't sure about what you are reading, you may want to look up the texts, and you'll retain more if you mark them.

Reviewers recommend re-reading this information because it's difficult to get the complex picture but it helps to look up and mark the texts to make them 'your own' in a 2nd reading.

In Daniel 8 there's a great horn on the goat that clobbers the ram. In Bible times, horns were used to make trumpets. Could the great horn represent Trump? It's looking like it could be!

When it comes to future events, we are a lot like the five blind men examining the elephant, each with a different report of what it's like.

If Christ were here today, He might say the same thing as He did then, but those phrases have different meanings now...

'<u>The time is fulfilled</u>'--is the 6,000 years that God gives us in the 4th Commandment. He gives us six days to work, but a day is like 1,000 years. Peter said not to be ignorant of it, 2Peter 3:8-10.

The previous verse (7) refers to things reserved unto fire for the day of judgment. Hawaii's fiery volcano and the unprecedented fires in California are shadows of what's coming...

We will see how papal visits intersected the jubilee timeline to signal the end of 1,000 years.

'<u>The kingdom of God is at hand.</u>' That's what the disciples wanted when they asked, 'Will you restore the kingdom to Israel at this time." Acts 1:6.

Christ's reply linked it to 'times and seasons' that Paul said we know--"for the day of the Lord comes as a thief in the night... for when they shall say 'Peace and safety,' sudden destruction comes." 1Thessalonians 5:1-3.

"Peace and safety' remind us of the Iran Nuclear Treaty or President Trump's Peace Plan for Israel and the Palestinians.

The good news in Noah's time was a boat--but they didn't believe it would rain and they didn't want to be laughed at. It takes faith to believe the Bible and see the good news in it. Christ said it would be "as the days of Noah." Matthew 24:37.

The good news for Abraham was the Promised Land. For Moses, it was freedom from bondage. Christ offered the spiritual aspect of freedom, but the Jews were more interested in getting rid of Romans.

The good news is better now, because it includes ALL of the above--all the great events of Bible history play a part in the grand climax that is building in the book of Revelation.

129

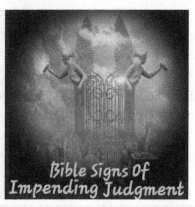

Bible Signs Of Impending Judgment

Judgment--Getting What We Deserve?

#1. Judgment can include getting what we deserve. This is sometimes called poetic justice, where the punishment matches the crime. In the end, we will all get what we deserve.

#2. But maybe not. In the Bible, God offers to forgive us if we repent with a change of mind and are sorry for our mistakes that the Bible calls sin, asking for His help to live better.

We are all guilty for causing the death of Christ and we need God's help to change so we live according to His Word.

His guidelines show us the way of life. They are the path to health and happiness, and He meets us more than half way.

Christ told a story of a wasteful son who asked for his inheritance before the father died--he was eager to see what the world was like and his dad was sad to see his son leave.

This prodigal son went to a far country and spent his money in riotous living. But like our world, things changed and a famine came.

To survive, this boy took a job feeding pigs and thought about of his father's servants eating better that he did, so he decided to go home and work as a servant for his father.

But his father was sensing his loss and watching for him. He ran to meet his son, illustrating God's love for us.

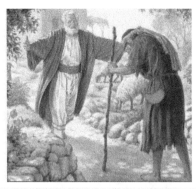

#3. In the Bible, the book of Judges shows that judges were deliverers. The name, Daniel, means God is my Judge, and God delivered him in Daniel chapters 1-6, in life-or-death situations because Daniel was willing to die rather than to do wrong or dishonor God--a huge lesson for us.

#4. The great thing about God is that He is not arbitrary. He leaves the choice to us. Our concept of God may cause us to run towards Him, seeing that He loves us and has a plan of salvation that goes far beyond our present problems...

Or the end-times may cause us to run from Him because we are bent on doing our own thing, or we can't believe in a God that loves us. Maybe He will burn us forever? Let's take a look at some common questions people have about God.

131

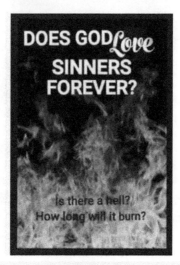

DOES GOD *Love* SINNERS FOREVER?

Is there a hell? How long will it burn?

Will God Love Sinners Forever in Hell?

That's what the devil might want us to believe. Who wants to love and worship a God that would delight in such torture?

This is a twisted teaching of the medieval church that developed the idea to get money! Just pay the priest to pray Mom or Dad out of purgatory or hell.

This is such a distorted view of God. Many are changing their minds about this idea. Let's look at what the Bible says.

Because the devil had accused God of being unfair and withholding from His creation a knowledge of all things, God allowed a test for Adam and Eve. If they were loyal to Him, they would live in that Paradise, but if they chose to disobey, they would die. He didn't say they would live in eternal torment, Genesis 3.

"The day comes, that shall burn as an oven; and all the proud, yea, and all that do wickedly, shall be stubble: and the day that comes shall burn them up, says the LORD of hosts, that it shall leave them neither root nor branch." Malachi 4:1

If this is so, why did Christ tell the story of the rich man and Lazarus which sounds like eternal torment?

It was a parable designed to teach that this life is all there is. It's like a time of probation to see if we will learn that God's way is best, or whether we are bent on doing our own thing...

The results of sin and a self-centered life that ignores the Giver is death for eternity, but God says, "I have no pleasure in the death of the wicked; but that the wicked turn from his way and live." Ezekiel 33:11.

To believe otherwise is to believe the devil's lies about a loving God that paid a painful price for our salvation.

We should rather believe what Matthew, Mark, Luke, John and Paul have written for us.

Another hard question about God is next...

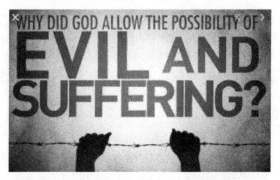

Why Does God Allow Evil and Suffering?

The Bible offers clues to how the angel, Lucifer, rebelled and became the devil--the source of evil.

"How are you fallen from heaven, O Lucifer... For you said in your heart, I will ascend into heaven, I will exalt my throne above the stars of God... I will be like the Most High." Isaiah 14:12-14.

But this wasn't just a private affair. He involved the angels of heaven and a third of them joined him in rebellion against God's government and were thrown out of heaven to earth. Revelation 12:7-9.

We might wonder, Why was he allowed to come to earth--why not zap him dead?

That's our human reasoning that plays into the picture that the devil paints of God, that He is stern and severe and demands our worship or He may strike us dead.

But since He doesn't kill the devil, millions think God is helpless--an absentee landlord of earth with all its woes.

But consider God's plight. If He pulled the plug on the devil and his angels (now called demons), all the other angels who didn't join Lucifer would not worship God from love, but fear that if they didn't tow the line, they would be gone too. That would mar the joy of serving God from appreciation for life and all that He gives us, which is how we should see Him.

"That the thoughts of many hearts may be revealed." In the light of the Saviour's life, the hearts of all, even from the Creator to the prince of darkness, are revealed. Satan has represented God as selfish and oppressive, as claiming all, and giving nothing, as requiring the service of His creatures for His own glory, and making no sacrifice for their good. But the gift of Christ reveals the Father's heart. It testifies that the thoughts of God toward us are "thoughts of peace, and not of evil." Jeremiah 29:11. It declares that while God's hatred of sin is as strong as death, His love for the sinner is stronger than death. Having undertaken our redemption, He will spare nothing, however dear, which is necessary to the completion of His work. No truth essential to our salvation is withheld, no miracle of mercy is neglected, no divine agency is left unemployed. Favor is heaped upon favor, gift upon gift. The whole treasury of heaven is open to those He seeks to save. Having collected the riches of the universe, and laid open the resources of infinite power, He gives them all into the hands of Christ, and says, All these are for man. Use these gifts to convince him that there is no love greater than Mine in earth or heaven. His greatest happiness will be found in loving Me." *Desire of Ages*, p 57.

As Einstein said, "It is better to believe than to disbelieve--in so doing you bring everything to the *realm of possibility*."

So it is for the "good news" Christ announced, and now we consider how "the time is fulfilled" in the next chapter.

135

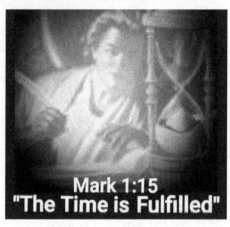

When Christ said, "The time is fulfilled," He was referring to the best-known time prophecy in the Bible. Daniel 9:24,25 points to Messiah, a word that means anointed.

But the Jews wanted deliverance from the Romans and missed the idea as Isaiah 53 gave His role to pay the penalty of our sin if we will appreciate His doing so and want to live on His side in the controversy with the devil who wants us to lose what God wants to give us if we appreciate Christ dying for us and we want to live by His guidelines that are for our best good.

70 weeks of years in Daniel 9:24 spanned 490 years with the Messiah coming one week (7 years) before the end of that prophetic period.

Christ was anointed by the Holy Spirit at His baptism, as described by John the Baptizer in John 1:29-34.

Those 70 sevens are foundational. They spanned 10 jubilees. Jubilee was defined as the 50th year in Leviticus 25:8-10, but the 50th jubilee comes to 1994-95 as explained next...

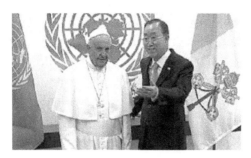

How Papal UN Visits Signal End-Times

God reinforced the weekly cycle of six days to work and the seventh day as a Sabbath that was made as a break for man's rest and it's said to be the Lord's day, Mark 2:27,28. In the yearly cycles, Israel was to rest the land every the 7th year.

After 7 sabbatical cycles (7 x 7 = 49), the 50th year was a Jubilee, but it came every 49 years because the 50th year was the 1st year of the next set of sevens.

In a jubilee year, debts were cancelled and Israelites were given freedom. If land had been sold, it came back to family ownership. A man could not sell his land and impoverish his children permanently. Leviticus 25:9,10.

The 490 years of Daniel 9 spanned 10 jubilees (49 x 10). They began with a jubilee event when Israelites were given freedom to leave Persia to get their land back in 457 BC. (Google Artaxerxes' decree, Daniel 9:25) The 70 sevens ended in 34 AD; both those dates were sabbatical years.

Fast-forward 40 more jubilees from the time of Christ (40 x 49 = 1960 years). Added to 34 AD, the 1960 years bring us to a sabbatical year in 1994 and the 50th jubilee in 1995 when Pope John Paul spoke to the UN on the Day of Atonement. That event fit Leviticus 25:9,10.

Then there was a 20 year gap until Pope Francis' UN visit, also on the Day of Atonement in 2015, but WHY a 20-year gap?

Peter says, "Be not ignorant, 1000 years are like a day, a day is like 1000 years...God is not slack...the day of the Lord will come." 2Peter 3:8-10.   137

If we integrate the jubilees into 1000 years, 10 jubilees of 490 years + 490 more = 980. There are <u>20 years left over</u>, **signaled by the popes' visits at the end!**

This suggests that papal visits at the end of the jubilee timeline marked the end of 1000 or 6000 years when the 7th millennium brings "the day of the Lord"—the end-time period and a time of judgment that Peter says not to ignore, 2Peter 3:7-10.

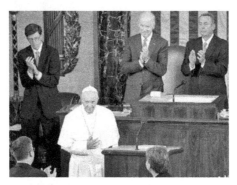

Five 'When-Then' Signs Also Marking 2015

For those who don't follow math as in the previous chapter, there were a series of 'when-then' signs that also marked 2015…

1."The day of the Lord was signaled by a rare solar eclipse on the equinox. It marked the same time as when God told Moses, "This *chodesh* (new moon crescent) is the beginning of the month, the first month of the year," Exodus 12:2.

If we go to Google images and type *chodesh, we* see it's the thin crescent moon that millions of people understand as the beginning of the new month (not the dark moon on the calendar).

Our Gregorian Calendar has no relationship between the new moon and new month and it is not the primary focus for biblical events.

2. Two weeks after the solar eclipse in 2015, there was a blood moon on Passover. This also is not common, and to have those two events marking the beginning of the biblical year in March, 2015 reminds us that "The sun shall be darkened and the moon turned to blood *before* the day of the Lord." Joel 2:31.

'Before' is from the Hebrew, *paniym;* it means facing the "day for the Lord." Those events faced end-times that are coming soon.

3."The day of the Lord comes as a thief; when they shall say 'Peace and safety,' sudden destruction comes" 1Thessalonians 5:2,3. Iran's Nuclear Treaty in 2015 was 'Peace and safety.' They have already violated it with missile tests.

4. Billy Graham said that God will have to apologize to Sodom if He waits longer to send judgment on the US. The Bible calls homosexuality an abomination in Leviticus 18:22, and it was 'standing where it ought not' (Mark 13:14) in the Supreme Court, adding to the 'when-then' signs like Christ gave about Lot fleeing Sodom, Luke 17:29.

5. Christ warned of the "abomination... <u>standing where it ought not</u>" in Mark 13:14. Early Christians understood his words as Rome and they fled when the Roman army came to Jerusalem in 66 AD. Doing so spared them the siege when Titus returned in 70 AD.

Rome was also "<u>standing where it ought not</u>" when the pope came to the US Congress because our Constitution says that Congress shall make no laws respecting the establishment of religion, but that's what the pope is all about. His *Laudato Si'* is about closing business on Sunday for family values and attending the Eucharist, paragraph 237 of an online pdf.

"Congress shall make no laws respecting the establishment of religion"--the 1st Amendment.

Respecting Sunday violates our Constitution and will allow the UN (image beast of Revelation 13:14-18 to compel false worship as the Bible predicts.

140

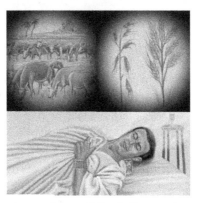

7 Good Years, Then 7 Bad Years, Genesis 41
Trump has been good for the economy

So where we are in the stream of time? We should be able to know--God won't do anything without revealing it, Amos 3:7.

"Teach us to number our days that we may apply our hearts unto wisdom," Psalm 90:12. We also find that God declares the end from the beginning, Isaiah 46:10.

In the book of beginnings, Genesis 41 offers insight. Pharaoh had two dreams and Joseph explained them. Seven fat cows were 'eaten' by seven lean cows that came after them.

Then seven heads of grain were full but nothing was left after seven thin heads of grain.

Joseph explained Pharaoh's dream as seven good years followed by seven years of famine and advised Pharaoh so wisely that Pharaoh appointed Joseph as prime minister to store the grain. Joseph saved Egypt!

The book of Revelation is said to integrate many historical events into the last seven years. "What is to come has been already, and God summons each event back in its turn," Ecclesiastes 3:15. Some Bible students see a 'twice speak' code. The fat cows and heads of grain support once in history and again for end-times.

Some scholars say the double imagery of fat and lean cows given again with heads of grain support a similar event for us.

141

There are a couple reasons why this may be so.

1. There were six days for Creation and then God rested or ceased His work. At the end of 6,000 years we may expect Christ to cease His work of mediation on a 7th year, a Sabbatical year that synchronizes with the Sabbatical year of 2015.
   Since the bad times haven't begun yet, we are in the 7 good years for the economy that could end with 2022, allowing end-times to begin in the spring of 2023. We will later see a 'heads up' sign for then.
2. The ceasing of Christ's intercession as our High Priest in a sabbatical year fits a 'chiastic' structure of the Bible. The end is a mirror image of the beginning.

As one goes down into a chasm and comes up and out the other side, we see man lost paradise in Genesis but has it restored in Revelation. The 7 good years in Genesis 41 enabled preparation for the 7 bad years. We should be preparing for what will break on the world as a huge surprise.

1. If the papal visits at the end of 50 jubilees and the 'when-then' signs in 2015 marked the end of 6,000 years* and

2. If the twice-speak code is a valid concept with "no slack," (2Peter 3:9) then the 7 good years began in 2016 and the 7 bad years and earthquake may be expected to start in 2023. "Teach us to number our days…" Ps 90:12.

Summary: 7 bad years in Daniel 4; 7 good years first in Genesis 41; 7 days for Jericho like Babylon--6 days with a trumpet each day (6 trumpets in Revelation 8 & 9) and 7 trumpets in the 7th day like 7 plagues in the 7th year, Revelation 16. This appeals to intuitive understanding with more to follow…

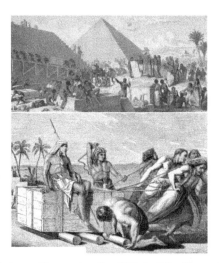

History Repeats: the US is like Egypt--
Killing Babies and Enslaving its People

Below are five examples of how the US is like Egypt at the time of the Exodus. Proud Egypt was humbled by calamity brought by God. History and Bible both warn us of impending judgment…

Paul said <u>the day of the Lord comes as a thief…</u> when they say 'Peace and safety,' sudden destruction comes on them <u>as travail on a woman with child.</u>" 1Thessalonians 5:1-3.

Egypt travailed with God's 1st-born, Exodus 4:22. We should see how the 7 good years in Egypt followed by 7 bad years are also for the US because the US has many parallels to Egypt.

1. Egypt was the strongest nation then as the US is the strongest nation now.

2. Egypt was the source of food in famine as America is for some nations now.

3. Israel went to Egypt in a time of famine as pioneers came to America in a time of famine for spiritual bread because the papacy banned the Bible—people hid it in their homes at the peril of their lives. They risked their lives at sea or starvation for freedom in the new world.

4. Another king came to power who didn't know Joseph. New pharaohs didn't recognize the rights and freedoms previously granted to Israel.

Like Pharaoh, many in Washington forget the Constitution gives freedom to citizens for self-government, but now federal government is huge and telling everyone what to do...

The principles of self-government came from the Bible. John Adams, our 2nd U.S. President said "the Constitution was designed only for a moral and religious people."

But after generations of TV's sex and violence, we are no longer "a moral and religious people."

5. Egypt killed babies and enslaved Israel. The US has aborted 60 million and has enslaved most of its population with alcohol, tobacco, caffeine and drugs that we call healthcare, but they're a leading cause of illness and death.

People are in bondage to food, fashion, fiction, gambling, greed, 'music,' sex, perversion, TV, movies, violence--a rainbow of negative lifestyles.

We're a nation in bondage by our choices and the Bible shows an impending time of judgment as when God executed judgment on Egypt and took Israel to a covenant agreement that made them His kingdom...

The good news is that God's kingdom is impending. God said, "If you will keep my covenant, you will be to me a kingdom," Exodus 19:5,6.

The only book Christ recommended to understand the end-times says that God will set up a kingdom 'in the days of these kings,' Daniel 2:44.

144

'The kingdom of God is at hand' Mark 1:15

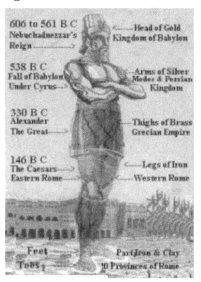

606 to 561 B C
Nebuchadnezzar's
Reign

Head of Gold
Kingdom of Babylon

538 B C
Fall of Babylon
Under Cyrus

Arms of Silver
Medes & Persian
Kingdom

330 B C
Alexander
The Great

Thighs of Brass
Grecian Empire

146 B C
The Caesars
Eastern Rome

Legs of Iron
Western Rome

Feet
Toes

Part Iron & Clay
10 Provinces of Rome

How God's Kingdom Will Be Set Up, Daniel 2

The above picture shows how easy it is for us to hear or see what we want to believe, because the picture is wrong!

Daniel 2:45 says the stone was cut out of the mountain without hands. What does that mean?

The only other usage of "mountain" in Daniel is Jerusalem--My holy mountain, but it represents God's people, and cut out without hands means no human devising. The pope or president of a denomination has no advantage over the wise virgins, (Christians who are ready), Matthew 25.

Everyone deserves an opportunity to hear and understand what we need to be part of God's kingdom for the end-time--just like in Egypt, there were Egyptians who left Egypt to be part of Israel. They were the "mixed multitude," Exodus 12:38.

And setting up the kingdom is *not* the 2nd coming. It's how God set up His kingdom at Sinai when He said, "If you keep my covenant, you will be to Me a kingdom." Exodus 19:5,6.

145

We saw the similarities of US with Egypt. God is going to execute judgment on the US. Those who are ready can be part of His kingdom.

Kingdom means dominion of a king. It's about His laws--the laws that Christ said are in effect "till heaven and earth pass." Matthew 5:18.

While it is true that we cannot earn our salvation by keeping the law, we shall not be approved by heaven if we don't want His guidelines.

"If you love Me, keep my commandments." They are not wild ideas--they make good sense and bring us peace, happiness and prosperity.

Israel's wisest king, Solomon said, "Righteousness exalts a nation." Proverbs 14:34.

Israel reached the peak of greatness under his reign when the major trade routes went through Jerusalem on the way to the India or China.

How surprised a heathen spy might have been if he could have crept into Jerusalem's Most Holy Place where the ark was, to discover the secret of Israel's greatness was not a gem-studded idol, but a law that defined our duty to God and others with equality and wisdom.

146

"Repent and Believe the Gospel"

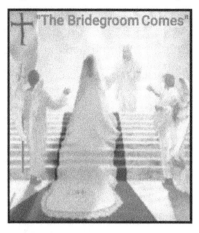

"The Bridegroom Comes!"

The Bible is God's love letter to us. He wants us to become familiar with it, "here a little, there a little" (Isaiah 28:10) so we know how it will fit together before it happens. He won't do anything without revealing it, Amos 3:7. We just need a greater familiarity with it, like pieces of a puzzle for the end-times, to put them together well.

The wedding parables reflect different aspects of what can be reality for us, but they seem so different that we miss what they have in common.

Luke's wedding parable is overlooked by most readers, but it is especially rich in helping us understand more. It's like the Rosetta Stone.

The Rosetta Stone was a discovery that helped to understand the Egyptian or hieroglyphics that were on a table of stone with the Egyptian and Greek languages.

Luke's wedding parable helps us especially the timing...

Passover is the Time of Judgment & Marriage

Luke's wedding parable with triple Passover imagery, and the cry at midnight in Matt 25:6 and Exod 12:29,30 make this at Passover--God won't do anything without revealing it, Amos 3:7

Passover was the historic time of judgment-- they were to pray for God to pass over them.

#1. "Have your loins girded." Luke 12:35. That phrase is first found at Passover, Exodus 12: 11

#2. "Watching" (*gregoreo*--be awake) is seen in Exodus 12:10 where Israel was awake and ate the Passover lamb, leaving nothing till morning.

#3. The Last Supper imagery in Luke 12:37 was also on the eve of Passover when Christ girded Himself and served His disciples as He promises to serve us if we are "watching."

Doing so is the key to high destiny, just as a woman's life changes if she marries a king!

The flip side of this is bad news for those who shrug this off. The servant who declines or fails to be watching will be beaten with stripes as Christ said in Luke 12:48.

Rapture thinking says God will not put His bride through tribulation, but the Bible says "we must through much tribulation enter the kingdom," Acts 14:22.

But the plagues fall on those who aren't sealed and haven't made a covenant as in Nehemiah 9:38.

The stripes for those who aren't sealed, Rev 9:4 and who accept the mark of the beast to go along with a New World Order, Revelation 13:14-18; 14:9,10.

And on the other hand, if we are winning in the conflict ahead, we probably won't mind because this promise is for us...

"Behold, I make a covenant (with you)...I will do marvels...I will drive out the Canaanite" Exodus 34:10,11.

We should see a parallel promise in the New Covenant that we may make. God says He will write His laws in our hearts so we want to do the right things. Jeremiah 31:31-33.

Without the New Covenant fulfilled to us, we wouldn't be safe to go to heaven. We might lust after someone and start trouble all over again.

We think not, but we don't even know our own hearts. "The heart is deceitful...desperately wicked," Jeremiah 17:9.

We can see this from Christ's letter to His last church. It is described as 'wretched, miserable, poor, blind and naked,' Revelation 3:17.

Why would Christ want to rapture this group to heaven? We have some growing to do!

God took Israel to the wilderness to prove what was in their hearts, and what they discovered wasn't good.

Egypt's history of watching at Passover and two wedding parables support our need to watch at Passover, the historic time of judgment, to be ready, but what does 'watching' mean?

149

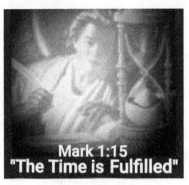

**Mark 1:15
"The Time is Fulfilled"**

Rapture Watch

The wedding parables of Matthew 25 and Luke 12:35-48 offer blessing and high destiny for those who are watching for Christ's coming, so we want to understand what He meant.

James and John wanted to be on His left and right hand in the kingdom. Christ asked if they could drink of His cup, which implies sharing what He would go through.

They said yes, and at the Last Supper, He gave them the cup, but hours later when He asked them to watch and pray, they slept. He said, "Could you not watch one hour?" Matthew 26:38-41.

It was the eve of Passover. Christians don't do Passover as Jewish people, but on the other hand, maybe we should eat the Lamb spiritually by reviewing the closing scenes of His life, thanking Him for taking our beating and praying to be more like Him.

'Blessed is that servant whom his Lord finds watching when He comes. He will gird himself and make him sit down to eat and will serve him,' Luke 12:37.

People think "watch" means to be aware, and everyone thinks they are aware. The Greek word, *gregoreo,* means to be awake. It would be unfair for Christ to tell us to be awake if there were no lues for when, because we can't be awake every night, but Passover was the only night it was commanded.

150

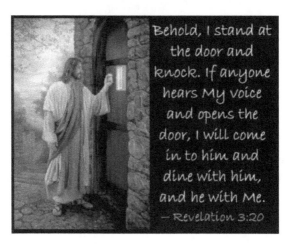

Behold, I stand at the door and knock. If anyone hears My voice and opens the door, I will come in to him and dine with him, and he with Me. — Revelation 3:20

"Open Unto Him Immediately" Luke 12:36
Christ is outside most US churches!

Luke's wedding parable (12:36,37) supports the idea that we must be watching to be ready because there is no later time to do so.

The women who came a little late were not admitted. The man with no wedding garment couldn't change and be back in a few minutes.

There will be no time later to get ready after a sudden unlooked-for calamity when the "day of the Lord" begins and God "shakes the earth mightily," Isaiah 2:21, New King James.

That earthquake is the "knock" in Luke 12:36 because the Bible explains itself, and the church of Laodicea where Christ knocked in Revelation 3:20 ended in an earthquake.

The earthquake is also as the "roar" of the Lion of Judah, Rev 5:5. It shakes the earth in Joel 3:16.

God won't do anything without revealing it and this includes His "roar" (earthquake) in Amos 3:7,8. Other passages have different imagery.

'The day of the Lord comes as a thief when they say Peace and safety, sudden destruction comes as travail on a woman with child, 1Thess 5:2,3.

151

Egypt travailed with God's first-born, Exod 4:22. The earthquake will bring travail to the US when end-times begin.

Another insight to 'open unto Him immediately' comes from the Rule of 1st Use. When Christ called James and John to follow Him, "they immediately left the ship and their father and followed Him," Matthew 4:22.

That was a huge opportunity for them, and so it will be for us. We should be willing to leave our ship (job) and close family ties if they are not supportive of our serving God in the end-time.

'Blessed is that servant whom his Lord finds watching--He will gird himself and make him sit down to eat and will serve him, Luke 12:37.

For the servant who is 'so doing when He comes He will make him ruler over all that He has,' Luke 12:44. This should be huge motivation...

And if we aren't "so doing," we will be beaten with stripes..."to whom much is given, of him much is required." Luke 12:48.

Think about this. This is so important to Christ that He is giving us the very highest incentive--to make us ruler over all that He has.

Being counted on His side when troubles begin can spare us 9/11 events. We all know 911 is about trouble. Christ's last six parables have a link to Numbers **9**:10,**11**, as it provides for when the end-times will begin with Passover timing in the 2nd spring month--knowing this, we can be watching as Christ asked His disciples, Matt 26:41

152

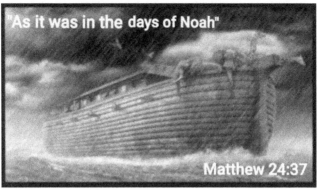

"As it was in the days of Noah"

Matthew 24:37

Big trouble coming!

The Flood brought an end to much wickedness and it came with Passover timing, but in the 2nd spring month as it fit one of Christ's six 9/11 clues that link to Numbers **9**:10,**11**.

We may think that's just an odd coincidence, but to students of Scripture, it's another example of God's infinite mind getting our attention with numbers that all Americans recognize and it implies that another 9/11 is coming!

Noah buried Methuselah, whose name meant, *at his death it will come.* He died as a sign that the Flood was imminent. Noah was unclean for contact with a dead body as the above text says.

The Flood came with Passover timing, but in the 2nd spring month. Noah entered the ark on the 10th day--that's when the Passover sacrifice was selected in Egypt, Exodus 12:3.

When people refused Noah's invitation, they selected themselves for sacrifice. God isn't arbitrary--He leaves the choice to us.

The good news was a boat--but it didn't seem like good news--they didn't think it would rain-- It takes faith to appreciate God's provision.

So it is now. There's a time of trouble coming "such as never was" (Daniel 12:1) and we would be wise to consider more of God's provisions before we are up to neck in alligators...

153

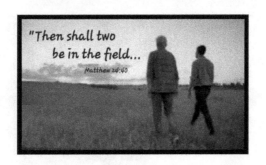

"Then shall two
be in the field...
Matthew 24:40

"Then shall two be in the field…" Matt 24:40
Was Christ talking about martial law?

"Then" means at the same time, or as an immediate consequence. The "9/11" timing in Numbers 9:10,11 for Noah's Flood might be ignored if it weren't for "then." But Christ's words got twisted into a fictional series of books and movies.

In the companion passage Christ said, "One shall be taken and the other left," the disciples asked, "Where, Lord?"

Christ replied, "Where the body is, there shall the eagles be gathered." Luke 17:37. Christ was not talking about a rapture--He was referring to the dinner of the birds in Revelation 19:17,18.

Christ's warning might mean martial law and being taken to a FEMA camp. "Being taken" isn't good. The parallel wording is the Flood came "and took them all away…"

Being taken could refer to those who don't heed Christ's warning to flee "when you see the abomination" that the early believers understood to mean the Roman army. They fled the city of Jerusalem and were spared the siege by Titus in 70 AD.

That was a type of end-times. The US military drill--JADE HELM (**H**omeland **E**radication of **L**ocal **M**ilitants), may have tested how a gun grab will work if we lose 2nd Amendment rights.

We would also lose 1st Amendment rights if Congress honors *Laudato Si'*, the pope's appeal for Sunday, but Sunday is a religious establishment, and is against the US Constitution. We need the US Constitution offering equal freedom to all.

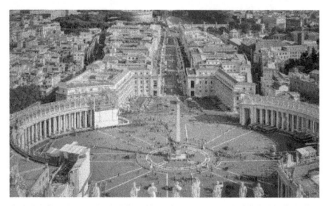

The Goodman, if he had known...would have watched and not suffered his house to be broken," Matthew 24:43.

The previous parables are linked to Passover timing in the 2nd spring month "as the days of Noah."

In the 2nd spring month at 2nd Passover, Pope Benedict went to Jerusalem in 2009. He didn't know it was 2nd Passover--it's not something observed by Jews now.

Most Jews have no interest in Moses' laws, nor do Christians, in spite of Christ saying, "Till heaven and earth pass, not one jot or tittle shall pass from the law, till all be fulfilled." Matthew 5:18.

If it wasn't important, why do Christ's closing parables all have links pointing to those times?

In Leviticus 23:44 they are called *mo'ed*. The word comes from Genesis 1:14 when God appointed or set times by sun and moon at the foundation of the world.

Christ is the Lamb, slain from the foundation of the world, Revelation 13:8. Those times foretold when it would happen.

More on this later, but it's significant that Pope Benedict proved to be the goodman in Christ's parable. How so?

The King James Bible only has one reference to the goodman in the Old Testament. It's in Proverbs 7:19,20 where a harlot tells a man, The Goodman is not at home; he is gone a long journey...and will come home at the *yom kece* (full moon)

Passover comes on a full moon, but "long journey" is a clue for 2nd Passover because Israelites didn't travel in winter, and if they took a long trip in spring and couldn't get back for Passover, they were to keep it a month later because of the provision in Numbers **9**:10,**11**.

It is not clear how to understand the full picture. Was Pope Benedict's house (pontificate) broken because he was on a long journey and didn't know when to watch?

Popes are married in a spiritual sense to the church and many Protestants believe his church is represented by the harlot in Revelation 17--so that would also fit the text of Proverbs 7:19,20.

This information isn't against so many fine Catholic Christians who live well and don't know what the leaders and secret societies of their church are doing to take control of America and make the pope head of a UN New World Order.

The pope will move to Jerusalem in the end-times as Daniel 11:45 suggests, to be in charge of the holy places for Jerusalem to be the international capital of the world.

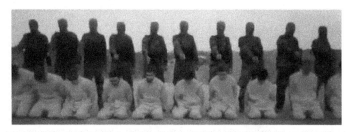

'Then shall the evil servant…smite his fellow servants'

The picture shows Muslim intolerance of Christians, but it fits the papal intolerance to Protestants for centuries as foretold in Daniel 7:25 and Revelation 17:6.

If we think we are so enlightened and tolerant now, Rwanda should jolt us to reality. A million Protestant Tutsis were slaughtered in spite of so many UN vehicles on the streets of Kigali, that "if you spit, you would hit one."

But the UN was ordered to 'stand down' and let the local (Catholic) government handle it.

John Paul later said 'sorry.' But prophecy for end-times shows many martyrs by guess who?

It could begin with Homeland Security (called Romeland Security by a former nun) rounding up patriot dissidents under martial law if they favor Bible prophecy over a UN New World Order--global democracy led by the pope, as in Revelation 17:3.

Daniel 12:1,7 shows a time of trouble such as never was when God's people will be scattered.

Christ's last night was a microcosm of end-times when He cited Zechariah--"Smite the shepherd and the sheep will be scattered," Matthew 26:31. The religious leaders were smiting Christ--They gave Him to Rome for execution.

"What is to come has been already, and God summons each event back in its turn." Ecclesiastes 3:15, NEB.

There's no 9/11 timing in this last parable of Matthew 24 but the next word is "Then…" (Same timing and that next parable is again like Numbers **9**:10.**11**.)

157

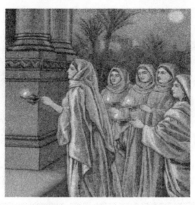

"Then shall the kingdom...be like 10 virgins"

Five of the 10 going to the wedding arrived too late and could not get in. Let's look closely at the meaning of Christ's words.

He said, "Watch," a clue for Passover as the only night that watching was commanded, Exodus 12:10.

Christ renewed this focus when He said, "Watch with Me--could you not [be awake] one hour?" Matt 26:38-41. They fell asleep and failing to pray, were unready for events that came suddenly. They scattered as He foretold.

We sometimes think they were stupid, but as a wise Master, Christ chose the best men available. They understood Passover as a likely time of judgment for the things that He was describing in Matthew 24.

But then He said, You don't know... It's a poor translation for the Greek *eido* that means to be aware, consider, understand.

Christ was saying, You don't understand and He explained why-- "for the kingdom is like a man traveling to a far country," Matthew 25:13,14.

If Israelites took a long journey in spring and couldn't get back for Passover, they were to keep Passover a month later, as shown again in **9/11** (Numbers **9**-10,**11**).

This is the 5th parable with a 9/11 link. Now comes #6

**"For the kingdom...is like a man traveling to a far country."
Matthew 25:14**

Most casual readers think Christ was merely changing the subject
to His last parable and fail to see this 9/11 link because they are
unfamiliar with the law that Christ said is in effect "till heaven
and earth pass," Matthew 5:18.

Christ's invisible return from a far country, (heaven) to execute
judgment in a parallel event as God did in Egypt, will catch most
people unready, for the day of the Lord comes as a thief when
they say 'Peace and safety.' 1 Thess 5:2,3

It comes down to our taking Him at His Word that is clear enough
if we are looking for His return. In this last parable, the wise
stewards were ready--only the lazy one was unready and he lost
the talent that he had been given.

More on readiness later, but one more parable supports end-times
to begin in late spring...it's about the fig tree.

159

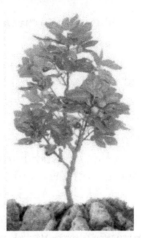

"Learn a parable of a fig tree...when summer is nigh"

Christ's words in Matthew 24:32 are probably not about Israel replanted since 1947 or 1967, and as said earlier, most Jews in Israel have no interest in their spiritual heritage.

Christ was probably referring to the fig tree that He cursed a couple days earlier because it was pretentious.

It was characteristic of the fig tree in that locality to have fruit when it had leaves, but this one, full of leaves, disappointed Christ--it had no fruit.

It was like the Jewish nation then, but it has a lesson for Americans now. Though established as a Christian nation, we are worse than Egypt with 60 million abortions and bondage to substances and negative lifestyles.

160

The Wedding Parables Are Not Understood

In Luke's wedding parable, Peter asked, "Is this parable for us, or for all?" Luke 12:41.

In Matthew 22, the King makes a marriage for His Son and sends His servants (this means us) to invite others to the wedding feast, but the invitation is scorned and messengers mistreated until the "remnant" get their city burned in Matthew 22:6,7. (King James Bible)

We might wonder why the invitation to the wedding was scorned, but if we remember the Passover setting, the scorners may prefer cake, steak and milk shake to a feast of unleavened bread at Passover, Leviticus 23:6.

But we should be thinking spiritually. It's not about crackers. Christ said, "Beware the leaven of the Pharisees," meaning their teachings in Matthew 16:12.

Churchmen have leavened the Bread (the Bible) by wanting to make it easy. For example, they say, You don't need to do Passover, but could we consider this...

"As Christ ate the Passover with His disciples, He instituted in its place the service that was to be the memorial of His great sacrifice." *The Desire of Ages,* pg 652.2

Doing the Lord's Supper on the eve of Passover (2nd month for reasons above), and then 'watch and pray' is the perfect way to be ready for end-times to begin as expected by His clues.

To be honest, I tend to fall asleep if I try to "watch and pray" as Christ said, but reading *The Desire of Ages* on the closing scenes of Christ's life and praying between chapters is a great spiritual exercise, even to include friends or neighbors.

"It would be well for us to spend a thoughtful hour each day in contemplation of the life of Christ. We should take it point by point, and let the imagination grasp each scene, especially the closing ones. As we thus dwell upon His great sacrifice for us, our confidence in Him will be more constant, our love will be quickened, and we shall be more deeply imbued with His spirit. If we would be saved at last, we must learn the lesson of penitence and humiliation at the foot of the cross." *Desire of Ages,* pgs 83.4

I don't know anyone who does this each day, but why not an authentic service on the eve of 2nd Passover with time to meditate on what He bore for us--eating the Lamb in a spiritual sense?

This is the perfect preparation for Christ's knock in Luke's wedding parable--"[Be] like unto men that wait for their lord, when he will return from the wedding; that when he comes and **_knocks_**, they may open unto him immediately.

"Blessed are those servants, whom the lord when he cometh shall find watching: verily I say unto you, that he shall gird himself, and make them to sit down to meat, and will come forth and serve them." Luke 12:36,37.

The 'knock' is probably the earthquake that initiates end-times-- that's how the church of Laodicea ended, circa 63 AD. And if He knocks (earthquake), we need to do the wedding feast."

162

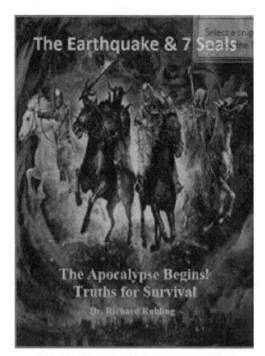

The Earthquake & 7 Seals

The Apocalypse Begins!
Truths for Survival

Dr. Richard Rubling

The Wedding Feast of Betrothal

The wedding feast at Passover is the Feast of Unleavened Bread, but it's not about crackers.

When Christ said to beware the leaven of Pharisees, He referred to their teachings, Matt 16:12. Church leaders leaven the bread, making it light, easy to swallow--no chewing needed.

The Feast of Unleavened Bread is different and we need to 'chew' it. It was a 7-day feast (Leviticus 23:6), like a week for Bible weddings, Genesis 29:27.

Those events coincide--they have the same meaning. Communion is union in the Word not leavened, and marriage is union by covenant based on the Word. There are seven topics for seven days of unleavened bread. They have a 7-fold emphasis in the Bible as a mark of end-time truth like the 7's in Revelation.

Here are a couple examples. Christ said before He comes, Elijah "must first come and restore all things." Matthew 17:11.

163

Elijah comes in the context of the statutes and judgments in Malachi 4:4,5. They have a 7-fold emphasis in Ezekiel 20:11-24-- they are linked to sabbaths as a sign of God's people.

The statutes, judgments and sabbaths are examples of topics to consider for a prenuptial feast of betrothal.

If we are faithful to our covenant for 7 years like Jacob was in his 7-year covenant before marriage, we can eat the wedding cake in heaven.

Another example from Genesis is the supper of betrothal when Rebekah made her decision to marry Isaac. As a miraculous birth and a willing sacrifice, Isaac was a type of Christ and Rebekah was a type of the 144,000, the spiritual bride of Christ that gets to follow Him wherever He goes in eternity, Revelation 14:4.

They are said to be 'virgins'--they must be the wise virgins that get in the wedding in Matthew 25:10.

Rebekah made the decision to marry a man she had never met at that supper. God doesn't want an ignorant bride for Christ--just as she listened intently, we must consider 7 topics that are a priority, indicated by their 7-fold emphasis for end-times, like the book of Revelation is a book of 7's for end-times.

When the disciples asked a sign for the end of the world, the first sign given was the destruction of Jerusalem in Matthew 24. So it may be like a 'heads up' for us when the 7 bad years are about to begin. Titus began his siege of Jerusalem in 70 AD at Passover. There are reasons why this repeat of history may be our sign...

164

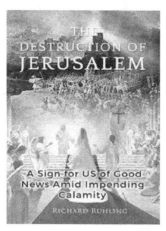

The Destruction of Jerusalem: a Sign for US

Christ said, 'When you see Jerusalem compassed with armies...its desolation is nigh," Luke 21:20

It happened in 70 AD--will it happen again? Yes! "The day of the LORD is coming and your spoil will be divided in your midst for I will gather all [Muslim?] nations to battle against Jerusalem; the city shall be taken, the houses rifled and the women ravished; half of the city shall go into captivity; Then the LORD will go forth and fight against those nations," Zechariah 14:1-3. There are wise reasons for this.

1. Most Jews in the land of Israel today have no interest in their spiritual heritage. Another group are Orthodox Jews who hate Christians. They are there because the UN gave them the land, but it wasn't the UN's land to give. It is God's land and after 50 jubilees--a time when land returns to the original owner (Leviticus 25:9,10) they are about to be chased out.

2. Their return to that land was premature. God said if they walk contrary to Him, that He would punish them 7 times over. Leviticus 26:18,21,28

For 390 years, they went contrary to Him, Ezekiel 4:5. They were taken captive by Assyria in 722 BC. 390 times 7 = 2730 minus 722 BC brings us to 2008, but with no year "0" it was 2009 when they would have been free to return. But in 2009, Pope Benedict went to Jerusalem and Christ warned believers to flee when they saw the abomination "standing where it ought not," Mark 13:14.

The pope represents abominations and seeing him in Jerusalem on the same year that the exiles could return was a heads up not to return if they understood Christ's warning.

Heeding His warning spared Christians in 70 AD and heeding His words now would spare Jews if they might reconsider their failure to count the 70 sevens of Daniel 9:24,25 to the Messiah, and the many prophecies He fulfilled, (see the Appendix.)

3. The war that will ensue from Zechariah 14:1,2 will bring an end to Muslim militancy in the Middle East, seen in Daniel 8, which Gabriel said is "at the time of the end." Daniel 8:17. For more info, see http://IslamUSinProphecy.wordpress.com

4. God says He will cause both Israel and Judah to return to the land that He gave their fathers, Jeremiah 30:3. Judah represents Jews who accept the Messiah and Israel represents the 10 tribes that were scattered among the nations and intermarried with Christians that also return, Jeremiah 31:10,16,17.

The reason that Jerusalem is "God's alarm clock" is because when we see Jerusalem "compassed with armies" (Luke 21:20) at Passover (historic timing for Titus' siege) we should expect judgment on the US a month later at 2nd Passover as explained. This would allow a similar time frame for *both* Israel and Judah to return and come together as dry bones after the shaking (earthquake) and get life as two sticks become one kingdom in Ezekiel 37:1-22.

166

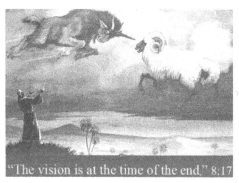
"The vision is at the time of the end." 8:17

A Muslim Ram & President Trump!

In Daniel 8, a militant Muslim ram angers a goat that flies from the west to stomp the ram and break its horns. The horns are said to be the kings of Medes and Persians in Daniel 8:20, but Gabriel said "the vision is at the time of the end," Daniel 8:17. Those areas are now Iraq and Iran.

The vision is half fulfilled with the death of Saddam. The next war is expected to be with Iran. Breaking the horn of Iran ends its militancy. Christians are spared by staying out of the war.

God "declares the end from the beginning." In the book of beginnings, Isaac was spared by sacrificing a ram, Genesis 22:13.

Muslims say Ishmael was the son that was spared by the ram. They celebrate the ram sacrifice each year--it's called Al-Adha.

Muslims should see the Bible is greater than the Quran because as Iran threatens to drive Israel into the sea, the horn (militancy) of Iran will be broken to spare Israel, son of Isaac, spared by the ram sacrifice in Genesis 22:13.

Note: Isaac was the father of Jacob whose name was changed to Israel in Genesis 32:28. We might see that Israel was spared when Saddam threatened them. The ram was caught in a **bush** in Genesis 22:13. The breaking of the ram's first horn (Saddam) came during the presidency of George <u>Bush</u>.

We should expect the breaking of the second horn (Iran) during the presidency of Donald Trump because animal horns were used to make trumpets. In Daniel 8:8, the goat that breaks the ram's horn has a great horn (Trump). After the horn of Iran is broken, the goat becomes "great," Daniel 8:8.

This is expected in the 2nd term, suggesting that Trump will win the election in 2020. The polls don't matter--remember Hillary!

It's amazing that Trump's campaign--Make America Great Again--may be seen in Daniel 8:8,17. Also interesting that hostility is shown against the message by Americans--it's almost like the devil doesn't want to see this prophecy fulfilled.

Jerusalem's destruction (previous chapter) may be the "heads up" sign of 'day of the Lord,' (Zechariah 14:1,2) before judgment falls on the US.

As Titus surrounded Jerusalem at Passover, we may expect similar timing for end-times when "all nations [Muslim] are gathered against Jerusalem," Zechariah 14:1-3.

They had a 'dry run' in April, 2018 as they gathered on the Gaza border for prayer. Attacking Jerusalem wouldn't make sense to us, but Muslim extremists don't need to make sense.

That would be the signal for judgment on the US a month later, at 2nd Passover for reasons seen previously.

"When you see Jerusalem compassed with armies" (Lk 21:20) we must give a 'midnight cry'--*the Bridegroom is coming,* (like when God judged Egypt and took Israel to a covenant, saying "I am married to you," Jeremiah 3:14.)

This includes readiness to come out of Babylon as Israel came out of Egypt. Coming out of the confused systems of this world represented by Babylon is the message in Revelation 18:2-4. Healthcare is one dimension already discussed...

168

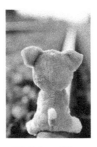

Education: Taking Your Children

Since kicking God out of the classrooms, the educational system has been getting worse with each decade and generation.

Parents naturally want the best for their children. It's an instinct, and it's a biblical thing.

If we take care of our children when they are small, they can reciprocate when we are old and need some help.

Rarely does a child have to do more for his parents than what they did for him growing up.

This is a biblical form of Social Security and it worked well in Bible times, but things change.

The government has intruded into the family circle and claims the right to take your child and teach what you may not appreciate, including sex education and perversion.

At the time of this writing, the state of Illinois is mandating LGBT education (Lesbian, Gay, Bisexual, Transgender). This is an abomination that could cause the land to spew us out. Leviticus 18:22,25. Hundreds now want to change back, sad...

If you love your children, get them out of the public schools that are doing so poorly. Most of education is not needed for life or work.

Having had 25 years of training to become board-certified in Internal Medicine and to teach on the university level, I would say that 90% of what I learned in college or medical school was not necessary.

That includes a chemistry major in college, calculus, physics, zoology, English literature, political science, history

Medical school was similar with a focus on anatomy, biochemistry and other topics that are mostly forgotten by graduation. We lose what we don't use.

Why not a system of apprenticeship under a competent person instead of book learning?

Another hazard of public schools now is the requirement of vaccinations and shots that are risky to one's health.

The Bible says, "Thou shalt teach them." Deuteronomy 6:7. That's how Christ learned. The schools of His time He did not seek...

170

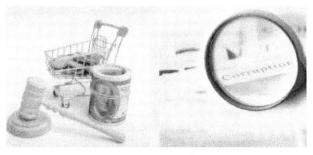

Bad Government

From the FDA that fails to regulate drugs as they accept money from drug companies and are soft on Monsanto and GMOs, we should know that most legislators are sold out and it's only a matter of time before America is gone.

This might also be understood from the CDC owning patents on vaccines so there are mixed motives for them telling us that we need to vaccinate our children--click for previous comment.

9/11 is another example. 1000 engineers have signed a document that jet fuel could not melt the steel beams of the World Trade Center.

What should we think of Defense Secretary, Donald Rumsfeld announcing $3.4 Trillion lost in the Pentagon budget the night before 9-11?

It never made headlines the next day--a missile (plane?) hit the accounting dept, no follow up could be done! If we think this was done by Muslims trained on small planes in Florida, we could be badly deceived.

171

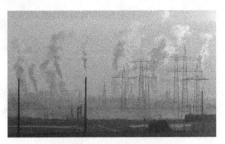

Leaving Babylon…the Cities

From the days of Lot in Sodom to the present, cities have been a focus of crime and immorality. Men left the farms for a 9-5 job but it's been downhill since then. It's a false economy as the agricultural base has shrunk and fewer people raise their food.

Millions now flock to the cities for welfare and housing. Government is bankrupt for answers. Cities are considered like 'deathtraps' by some. Joel Skousen's *Strategic Relocation* is about survival in areas of low population density. All of this fits the Bible message, Babylon is fallen, come out…

If We Fight, We Die in the Coming Civil War

Yes, godly men fought for this country and braved death to establish its freedom in 1776. But contrary to what many believe, the clock can't be turned back to 1776. We hate what we see happening to America–there's been too much "change" that millions wanted and voted.

Colonel Ammerman (under Gen. Schwarzkopf in Desert Storm) cited unclassified information to say there were a million UN troops in North America, mostly on closed military bases (more than a decade ago, so you might double it).

Department of Defense Confirms Russian Troops To Train On U.S. Soil. Although this is the first time Russian troops will train on U.S. soil, soldiers from other nation have done so for more than a decade.

Perhaps this is because they won't hesitate to shoot US citizens when US troops with concern for the Constitution, (already with a high suicide rate) might have a problem with that.

"History repeats" and the following parallel should be instructive to us. When Israel failed to honor God as America has, God allowed the Babylonians to take them captive. The prophet, Jeremiah, said, _If you resist, you will die,_ "but he that goes out and falls [surrenders] to the Chaldeans that besiege you, he shall live." Jeremiah 21:9.

Paul included the Exodus when he said, "All those things happened for examples... ends of the world," 1Corinthians 10:1,11. Christians don't understand, and Christ said the invitation to the marriage would be scorned, Matthew 22:3-6.

"If you are Christ's, you are Abraham's seed and heirs according to the promise [of land]" Galatians 3:29. When New World Order is set up and you can't buy or sell without being compelled to worship falsely (Revelation 13:15-17), the land of the covenant that God made with Abraham will be the only place for true Christians. Going to Israel is also the context of the New Covenant Promise to write His laws in our hearts, Jeremiah 31:8,10,17,31.

It's an awesome thought. That's the last place we might like to go now, but after Zechariah 14:1-3 when God begins to fight against those nations, it will be safe to go, also promised in Ezekiel 36:24-28–"I will take you from among the heathen (America is getting that way!) and gather you out of all countries and will bring you into your own land. THEN (we get a new heart and right spirit without which we will not be ready to meet Christ in the sky)...and you will dwell in the land that I gave your fathers (hint–it's not about America anymore!)

We might not want to go there, but there really isn't any choice because it's the land of the covenant, promised by God to Abraham's seed, and "If ye be Christ's, then are ye Abraham's seed and heirs according to the promise [of land]" Galatians 3:29.

When the whole world is under New World Order and can't buy or sell without false worship (Revelation 13:15-17) they will receive the wrath of God, Revelation 14:9,10--then God will defend His covenant-keeping people in the land of the covenant.

173

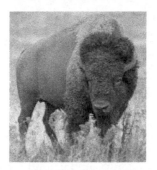

Roots and How History Repeats

The Founding Fathers understood many of the biblical principles we've mentioned, and they wisely crafted a constitution that maximized freedom of individuals while minimizing the power of government.

But as President John Adams said, "Our Constitution was made only for a moral and religious people. It is wholly inadequate to the government of any other."

Many early Americans understood that the sea beast in Revelation 13:1-10 was the papacy that they had fled. Its 'deadly wound' was the Protestant Reformation, and now that wound is healed as foretold, seen by Lutherans having joint communion with Catholics to end 500 years of division.

Some early Americans saw that the 2nd beast in Revelation 13 represented the US. The two uncrowned horns pictured above, represent a government without a king and a church without a pope—Protestant America.

But a change occurs and this 2nd beast makes an image—a look-alike to the 1st beast (papacy). The United Nations is the image beast and it will look like the papacy when the pope is asked to be in charge. Being in charge is supported by the imagery of the harlot riding the beast in Revelation 17:3.

A friend asked a Mexican couple why they moved to Montana. They replied, "Because the priest told us to…" Catholics have strategized to outmaneuver other voting blocks in gaining control of most local governments.

"When the time comes and men realize that the social edifice must be rebuilt according to eternal standards, be it tomorrow, or be it centuries from now, the Catholics will arrange things to suit said standards.

"They will make obligatory the religious observance of Sunday on behalf of the whole of society and for its own good, revoking the right of free-thinkers and Jews to celebrate incognito, Monday or Saturday on their own account. Those whom this may annoy, will have to put up with the annoyance.

"Respect will not be refused to the Creator nor repose denied to the creature simply for the sake of humoring certain maniacs, whose frenetic condition causes them stupidly and insolently to block the will of a whole people." *The Liberal Illusion,* Louis Veuillot, published by the National Catholic Welfare Conference, Washington DC.

Rome admits that there is no biblical authority for Sunday worship—it is on the basis of their church authority. This will bring "Protestants" to a test of their "Sola Scriptura" that they claim is the basis of their faith.

When the US accepts UN sovereignty, the pope will get his 42 months as foretold in Revelation 13:5.

Books that support this information would include books on the history of the reformation, "Rome Stoops to Conquer," "The Godfathers," and "The Great Controversy"--these may be found on Amazon or by Googling above titles, some available in pdf.

Summary

In this book we have looked at a broad picture of Scripture for end-times. We have seen that the US is worse than Egypt that killed babies and put Israel in bondage, and we have negative lifestyles worse than Egypt. The US is overcome by false systems of healthcare, education, government and religion. (more below)

God is going to "execute judgment" (Exodus 12:12) as He did on Egypt and those who are 'watching,' Lk 12:37 on the eve of

2nd Passover as per Christ's 9-11 clues in his last parables, will be blessed with an opportunity to become the Bride of Christ for purposes beyond the scope of this book.

In Matthew 25, the cry at midnight (sudden calamity in Exodus 12:29,30) was the signal for the wise to put extra oil in their lamps and go to the wedding. *The Earthquake & 7 Seals* is the oil that we need to find the wedding--7 topics that are the basis for a prenuptial covenant, like Jacob was betroth to Rachel for 7 years--it's 7 years for us.

The 7 topics have a 7-fold emphasis in the Bible as a mark of end-time truth, like the book of Revelation has 7 seals, trumpets, thunders, etc. You can get *The Earthquake & 7 Seals* on Amazon (click the link), or my website below. God bless you!

"It's more blessed to give than to receive," Acts 20:35. So often we think it means money, but what about the blessing of sharing the message with others? We can be the King's servants to bid others to the wedding (Matthew 22) if we choose to do so, and in the parable of Luke 12:35-44, "He will make [us] ruler over all that He has" if we meet the conditions that include having our lights burning…how hard is that?

As the title of this book says, Health, Happiness and Destiny come from wise choices--follow me to a better life! At 77, my health, happiness and destiny are the essence of life and more valuable than gold, but they come from wise choices that you can make and have them as well.

Please visit http://richardruhling.com for added materials, and I think you will also like the topics in the appendix…

Appendix

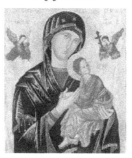

For Catholics

God loves everyone and there are many fine Catholic Christians who live up to all the light that they have and are therefore, better off than many Protestants who don't.

We cannot categorize everyone by the church they attend, but as a rule, the Catholic Church does little to educate its members in the Bible, though they are taught the catechism.

Sadly, some of the catechism is just plain wrong, even with things as basic as the Ten Commandments.

If you are Catholic, you might be surprised to compare the 10 Commandments in Exodus 20 of a Catholic Bible with your catechism. (Exodus is the next book after Genesis.)

The 2nd Commandment forbids the use of images, but the church is full of them, so the catechism got rid of that commandment, and to maintain ten commandments, the 10th was divided into two—You shall not covet your neighbor's wife, and You shall not covet his things.

But the Bible does not allow changes to be made, Deuteronomy 4:2 and the church also changed the Sabbath that God gave as a memorial of Creation when God ceased His work on the 7th day, Genesis 2:2,3 and Exodus 20:8-11.

Sunday, the day of pagan sun worship is now honored. It comes from the Edict of Constantine in 321 AD, in an effort to unite his empire.

All of this and more was foretold by God in Daniel 7 where a little horn would grow out of the 4th beast that represented the Roman Empire.

Protestant reformers saw that little horn represented the papacy that persecuted them. It changed times and laws and spoke blasphemy claiming to be the vicar of Christ. One of his titles is "Lord God the Pope."

Millions of Catholics have little or no understanding of Bible truth or how to be saved. The priest claims to forgive sin and offer salvation, but the widespread pedophilia supports their not being included in the 7 churches of Revelation 2,3 to whom it is said, "To him that overcomes, will I give…"

Rome does not have a system of belief that helps people to overcome sin, and the priests are morally bankrupt.

Christians understand that when they give their life to Christ, He saves them from the penalty AND the power of sin so that they have a new heart and want to do His will.

After a description of Babylon (another name for the papacy in Revelation 17), there's a call to come out of Babylon, and be not partakers of her sins and receive not of her plagues, Revelation 18:4.

For an excellent guide on how to know Christ as your personal Savior, you can read a great book that is translated into more than 100 languages and it's non-denominational at
https://bit.ly/2lAHhPT

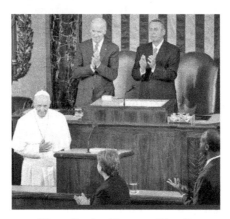

How Is the Pope a Sign?

In 66 AD, the Roman army represented an abomination "standing where it ought not…" Mark 13:14.

In 2015, Rome's leader was also *standing where he ought not* when the pope came to Congress, but most people wouldn't understand it without some history.

Historians say 50-100 million were martyred in the Holy Roman Empire when kings did the pope's bidding against heretics, defined as those who wouldn't bow to the pope. One of his titles is "Lord God the Pope." (Google)

The Bible represents God's people as a woman, Jeremiah 6:2. Speaking of the church, "The woman fled into the wilderness where she had a place prepared of God," Revelation 12:6.

Pioneers risked their lives at sea and from Indians or starvation, but God helped them. And they made a wise Constitution that was like the Ten Commandments--it was mostly about self-government, but things have been changing.

*In Pope Pius IX's 'Syllabus of Errors' that are **part of the ordination vows of priests worldwide**, we read their intent for world supremacy that includes the conquest of America's Constitution:*

15. "No man is free to embrace and profess that religion which he believes to be true, guided by the light of reason."

17. "The eternal salvation of any out of the true church of Christ is not even to be hoped for."

18. "Protestantism is not another and diversified form of the one true Christian religion in which it is possible to please God equally as in the Catholic Church."

21. "The Church has power to define dogmatically the religion of the Catholic Church to be the only true religion."

24. "The Church has the power of employing force and (of exercising) direct and indirect temporal power."

37. "No national Church can be instituted in a state of division and separation from the authority of the Roman Pontiff."

42. "In legal conflict between Powers (Civil and Ecclesiastical) the Ecclesiastical Law prevails."

45. "The direction of Public Schools in which the youth of Christian states are brought up... neither can nor ought to be assumed by the Civil Authority alone."

48. "Catholics cannot approve of a system of education for youth apart from the Catholic faith, and disjoined from the authority of the Church."

54. "Kings and Princes [including, of course, Presidents, Prime Ministers, etc.] are not only not exempt from the jurisdiction of the Church, but are subordinate to the Church in litigated questions of jurisdiction."

55. "The Church ought to be in union with the State, and the State with the Church."

57. "Philosophical principles, moral science, and civil laws may and must be made to bend to Divine and Ecclesiastical authority."

Roman Catholicism, Dr. Loraine Boettner, Presbyterian & Reformed Publishing Co. pdf here, https://bit.ly/2jZGNCL

Rome has conquered the US. Washington DC is surrounded on three sides by Mary-land.

The CIA is Catholic Intelligence Agency or Catholics In Action (Google). Homeland Security is called Romeland Security by a former nun who left the church after a priest raped her.

The pope's visit to Congress with his *Laudato Si'* encyclical uses a debatable cause, global warming, as a basis for legislation to close businesses on Sunday to reduce greenhouse gases and have a day for family values and the blessings of the Eucharist.

But "Congress shall make no laws respecting an establishment of religion..." 1st Amendment to the Constitution. Is it really needed?

NOAA/NCEI annual global analysis for 2018:

"Overall, the global annual temperature has increased at an average rate of 0.07°C (0.13°F) per decade since 1880 and at an average rate of 0.17°C (0.31°F) per decade since 1970. The 2017 average global temperature across land and ocean surface areas was 0.84°C (1.51°F) above the 20th century average of 13.9°C (57.0°F), behind the record year 2016 (+0.94°C / +1.69°F) and 2015 (+0.90°C / +1.62°F; second warmest year on record) both influenced by a ***strong El Niño episode***. The year 2017 is also the warmest year without an El Niño present in the tropical Pacific Ocean."

Global warming is not the problem--it's the hurricanes that can be blamed on "a little know Pentagon project" reported in *Popular Science,* Sept, 1995. It showed an acre of microwave towers in Alaska that beam high energy into the ionosphere to be reflected into the ocean, heating it up to cause El Ninos. It's called HAARP --High Altitude Aurora Research Project...

181

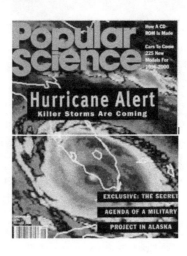

The article said it's "a little known Pentagon project." Please connect the dots--Pentagon...CIA...Catholics In Action (Google) because its leaders are members of Catholic secret societies like Knights of Columbus, Knights of Malta, Opus Dei, etc.

Their allegiance is to the pope and his agenda for *Laudato Si'* and Sunday (paragraph 237, online pdf) which is against the US Constitution. A civil war seems likely. The pope rides the beast (government) of a UN New World Order in Revelation 17:3, but Mother Miriam (nun) says the "pope's new humanism would wipe out Christianity." (YouTube). Lots of Catholics are concerned...

"When the time comes and men realize that the social edifice must be rebuilt according to eternal standards, be it tomorrow, or be it centuries from now, the Catholics will arrange things to suit said standards...They will restore Jesus to His place on high, and He shall no longer be insulted. They will raise their children to know God and to honor their parents. They will uphold the indissolubility of marriage, and if this fails to meet with approval of the dissenters, it will not fail to meet with the approval of their children. They will make obligatory the religious observance of Sunday on behalf of the whole of society and for its own good, revoking the permit for freethinkers and Jews to celebrate incognito, Monday or Saturday on their own account. *The Liberal Illusion,* Louis Veuillot, published by the National Catholic Welfare Conference, Washington, DC.

All of the above is based on an understanding of Revelation 13, and it was predicted by my favorite author, Ellen White, whose health and happiness sections of this book is huge because they were published more than 100 years ago and are in the public domain now.

Her book, *The Great Controversy,* is a classic that reads like the evening news. Here's a paragraph that fits the above info on hurricanes from the HAARP project in Alaska…

"While appearing to the children of men as a great physician who can heal all their maladies, he will bring disease and disaster, until populous cities are reduced to ruin and desolation. Even now he is at work. In accidents and calamities by sea and by land, in great conflagrations, in fierce tornadoes and terrific hailstorms, in tempests, floods, cyclones, tidal waves, and earthquakes, in every place and in a thousand forms, Satan is exercising his power. He sweeps away the ripening harvest, and famine and distress follow. He imparts to the air a deadly taint, and thousands perish by the pestilence. These visitations are to become more and more frequent and disastrous." *The Great Controversy,* pg 589.

The book was advertized in *TIME Magazine* for $21.95 plus postage but a well-illustrated 90-page condensation is available for $3 at http://richardruhling.com/donate.aspx (Option 3) or you get it as a free bonus if you donate $10 for the dvd (Option 1) that you'll love, also at this link…

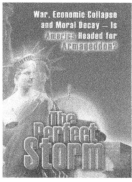

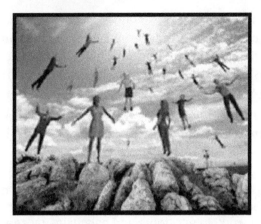

Problems for a Pre--Tribulation Rapture

1. There's a biblical precedent of God <u>executing judgment on Egypt</u>, taking Israel to a **covenant** that He **regarded as a marriage**.

He said, Return to Me--I am married to you, Jeremiah 3:14. Paul included the Exodus in "**all those things happened to them for our examples**...ends of the world, 1Cor 10:1,11.

2. We aren't ready for heaven. The last church is described as materialistic and lukewarm, with Christ outside knocking for entrance. Blind and naked aren't great attributes, Revelation 3:17. Why would God rapture us to heaven when we have some growing to do?

3. "We must through much tribulation enter into the kingdom..." Acts 14:22. Saying that God won't put His bride through trouble is forgetting that He took Israel to the wilderness to prove what was in their hearts, and it wasn't good. "The heart is deceitful...who can know it?" Jer 17:9.

4. The rapture occurs when "we shall all be changed...<u>at the **last** trumpet</u>" 1Cor 15:51,52.

There are 7 trumpets in Revelation 8:5,6 that are preceded by an earthquake that shakes the earth to initiate the end-times, Isaiah 2:21; Joel 2:10,11

5. "Rapture texts" are often out of context as we saw when one is taken and the disciples asked, Where, Lord? He replied, Where the body is, there will the eagles gather, Luke 17:36,37.

Those words of Christ are not a pre-tribulation rapture, but they might mean being taken to a FEMA camp for New World Order screening and re-education. Those preferring a biblical understanding in Revelation may face death like Daniel and his friends in Daniel 1-6.

Some scholars are no longer convinced on the rapture, and it's too easy to jump to conclusions when something isn't clearly taught in the Bible.

For example, Christ says that "when He comes and knocks," we should "open to Him immediately." Luke 12:36.

If you have been taught to believe in a rapture, it may be easy to think that's what Christ means here. But several points don't fit rapture teaching.

Why would Christ say, "Have your loins girded, have your lights burning" if He were going to rapture us, even from sleep? We don't need to sleep with our clothes or lights on. This is about something else.

Here are some additional considerations:

1. Christ said, "As in the days of Noah," Luke 17:26. Noah wasn't raptured; he came through the storm. Enoch was raptured before Noah was even born, so his being taken to heaven had nothing to do with avoiding the Flood or tribulation.

3. Elijah was raptured, but Christ never said the end would be like Elijah for us. Elijah was raptured only after he confronted false worship of Baal. Our confrontation will be with Antichrist when the United Nations mandates everyone to be marked or implanted for identity purposes, for this will be contrary to the Bible, Revelation 13:16,17; 14:9,10.

4. "As it was in the days of Lot," Luke 17:28. Lot wasn't raptured. He was told to flee, and Christ told us to flee because there would be great tribulation, Matthew 24:15-21; Mark 13:14-20. 185

5. Everyone else in history has faced trouble and death. "Now all these things happened unto them for examples, and they are written for our admonition, upon whom the ends of the world are come," 1Corinthians 10:11.

6. When asked about the end of the world, Christ said to understand Daniel. The book of Daniel shows no rapture. Daniel and his friends were tested by a series of life or death situations. "Daniel" means God is my Judge and we may only be judged when we face death and do right. Otherwise we may be "fair-weather" Christians.

7. "By their fruits ye shall know them." The fruit of rapture teaching is a lack of Bible study in Revelation, thinking "we won't be around." But Revelation is the only book that Christ promises a blessing for reading it, Rev 1:3.

8. We would feel like second class citizens in heaven if we were raptured from trouble and lukewarm materialism (Revelation 3:17) if we did not have the opportunity to face trouble manfully as did Daniel, Peter or Paul.

If we are faithful through this refining process -- trumpet plagues of Revelation 8,9, the mark of the New World Order, Revelation 13:16,17 and the 7 vials that fall on those who receive that mark, Revelation 14:9,10--we will be ready to meet Christ when He comes visibly. "Every eye shall see Him, Revelation 1:7 and 19:11.

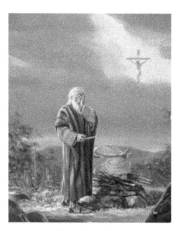

For Jews Seeking the Messiah

The sh'ma from Scripture says, "Hear, O Israel: The LORD our God is one LORD." Deuteronomy 6:4.

This argument against Christ being God's Son fails to see that the word for "one" is *echad*; and it means a combined unity as when the evening and morning became one day, and when a man "shall cleave unto his wife and they shall be one flesh, Genesis 2:24.

This suggests the Godhead are *echad*—a combined unity of divine beings who are one in character, one in purpose, all-knowing, and all-powerful.

This combined unity fits the Hebrew word for God, *elohim,* used 2605 times in the Bible, because "elohim" is the *plural* form of the word for God.

"And God [elohm, plural] said, Let us make man in our image," Genesis 1:26. Who was He talking to?

We should consider that Abraham (pictured above) was a type of our heavenly Father. Abraham was tested on the point of his willingness to sacrifice his son.

His answer to Isaac is classic—"God will provide Himself a lamb," Genesis 22:8. If we don't allow for this, we cannot understand the sacrificial role of the Messiah's first advent described in Isaiah 53—   187

"He is despised and rejected of men; a man of sorrows, and acquainted with grief: and we hid as it were our faces from him; he was despised, and we esteemed him not. Surely he has borne our grief, and carried our sorrows: yet we did esteem him stricken, smitten of God, and afflicted. But he was wounded for our transgression, he was bruised for our iniquities: the chastisement of our peace was upon him; and with his stripes we are healed. All we like sheep have gone astray; we have turned every one to his own way; and the LORD hath laid on him the iniquity of us all," Isaiah 53:3-6.

Asking questions about God, Solomon then asks, "What is His name and what is His Son's name, if you can tell?" Proverbs 30:4.

Moses' law says, "at the mouth of two witnesses, or at the mouth of three witnesses shall the matter be established," Deuteronomy 19:15.

Matthew, Mark and John were cowards that ran when Christ was taken, but were willing to die for Him after the resurrection. Two or three who saw Him are stronger evidence than a million who didn't see Him.

Matthew, especially, shows many of the prophecies concerning Christ were fulfilled by His birth, life and death. Psalm 22, for example, gives Christ's words on the cross and says His hands and feet were pierced, verse 16. Roman crucifixion was not invented until centuries later. Here's a video with 300 prophecies of the Messiah https://bit.ly/2kpTOpi

Sadly the Jews failed to see Daniel's 70 x 7 in Daniel 9:24,25. It resulted in a disaster for them when they said, "We have no king but Caesar," John 19:15. "His blood be on us and our children," Matthew 27:25. In Daniel 9:25,26, Messiah came _before _the destruction of Jerusalem in 70 AD. They missed Him! We need to be open to Truth in whatever guise it may come to us.

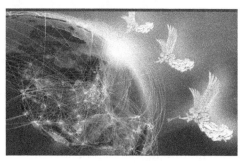

Seventh-day Adventists, Jehovah's Witnesses, Latter Day Saints & other Claims for Truth

The seven churches in Revelation 2 and 3 were not just in Asia Minor--they span the time from then till now; western Christianity today fits the last lukewarm church. We are too content with materialism while Christ is not in the church—He's outside knocking.

Christ said, "I am...the Truth," John 14:6. It is Truth that begs an entrance to churches today and the message of Revelation 3 addresses the *aggelos,* the messenger or preacher who is blind and naked, verse 17.

This means his loins are not girded with truth, Ephesians 6:14. This is especially true on the topic of the wedding parables because <u>there are seven parallels between Luke's wedding parable and Revelation 3:17-21</u> but not seen as such.

Both get a 'knock' and are to open. To sit with Christ on His throne (Rev 3:21) is the same as "ruler over all that He has," Luke 12:44.

God does not discriminate against any group. He is "not willing that any should perish, but that all should come to repentance," 2Peter 3:9.

The problem is with groups that think they have it all but they aren't like the Bereans who received the word with readiness and searched the Scriptures to see if those things were so." Acts 17:11

Seventh-day Adventists are an example with many preachers saying, We are not saved by works, we just need a relationship with Jesus. But He's outside the door (Revelation 3:20) and how can He save us if we don't do what He said?

Adventists grew out of the Great Disappointment in 1844 when a Baptist Wm Miller preached a rapture (2nd coming). Their experience may be seen in the 'bitter belly' experience of John in Revelation 10:10--he ate the little book. It was the book of Daniel because of similar imagery in Revelation 10 and Daniel 12.

The Angel with one foot on land and sea, denoting ownership was Christ. He said, You must prophesy again, but SDAs do not seem interested in doing so, afraid of another disappointment?

This book shows how we may be spared if we watch for the destruction of Jerusalem as the sign Christ gave in Luke 21:20 and it fits Zechariah 14:1,2. If we see that at Passover like when Titus began his siege in 70 AD, that is when we should "prophesy again" and give the message, 'the Bridegroom comes!'

It suggests a repeat of history as when God came to Egypt as Bridegroom and took Israel to a covenant (later saying, "I am married to you," Jeremiah 3:14) but He also "executed judgment" on Egypt and we saw earlier how the US is like Egypt.

History is going to repeat in a similar way. Millions of Christians think they are ready to be raptured, but we must have the New Covenant Promise of His law written in our hearts, and it has a 'latter day' context that we overlook in Jeremiah 31:1,8,17.

In Acts 7:52, Stephen asks, "which of the prophets did your fathers not persecute?" The implied answer is they were all perse-cuted. This applies to Ellen White that Seventh-day Adventists regard as a prophet, but they didn't follow her on numerous points, like their teaching of pharmacology at Loma Linda.

For Christians not familiar with her writings, an excellent book is *The Great Controversy* and a well-illustrated condensation of it, theperfectstormiscoming.org is the title and where to download it free. It explains What's Behind the New World Order? (same book)

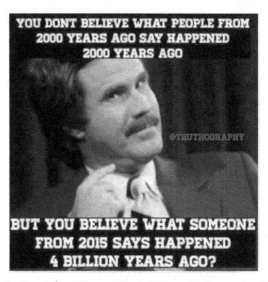

YOU DONT BELIEVE WHAT PEOPLE FROM 2000 YEARS AGO SAY HAPPENED 2000 YEARS AGO

@TRUTHOGRAPHY

BUT YOU BELIEVE WHAT SOMEONE FROM 2015 SAYS HAPPENED 4 BILLION YEARS AGO?

Evolution? Leading Atheist Now Believes in God

An Oxford University philosophy professor, Antony Flew, who has been a leading champion of atheism for a half-century has changed his mind. He now believes in God. (Google)

Biologists' investigation of DNA "has shown, by the almost *unbelievable complexity* of the arrangements which are needed to produce life, that **intelligence must have been involved**," Flew says.

What Flew is saying about DNA complexity could apply to other fields of science. Almost without exception, astronomers who study the complexity of the universe see intelligent design and believe in a super-intelligence.

The 2nd Law of Thermodynamics [Entropy] says that the energy systems of the universe run down unless acted on by an outside force. This is why a scientist said it would be easier to believe a jumbo jet resulted from an explosion in a junkyard than for life to have evolved on earth after a "Big Bang." *TIME Magazine.*

How would evolutionists explain this? "May 5, 2000: The date that Mercury, Venus, Mars, Jupiter and Saturn will line up with the sun and moon—the first time in 6,000 years." *TIME Magazine* Jan 17, 2000.

The "Big Bang Theory" of an explosion would send fragments in all directions. How would orbiting of nicely rounded spheres occur at a 6,000 year interval that signifies time is up for earth because after six days of creation, God ceased His work (Genesis 2:2) and 1,000 years are as a day, 2Peter 3:7,8.

This explains the solar system alignment as a sign that time is up and we are entering a time of judgment. Since 2000 many things are beginning to unravel, including 9/11 as a marker.

But if God is really the Author behind the Bible, we should expect it to reflect "intelligent design" like the solar system alignment or the complexity of DNA.

And, indeed, it does have intelligent design. And there are scores of difficult questions that evolutionists are unable to answer that required all steps of evolution to evolve simultaneously or it wouldn't work --like the cascade of reactions for clotting of blood so a minor cut or trauma doesn't cause one to bleed to death.

The development of vision in our eyes is another example. A mouse trap can't evolve; all parts are needed at once or it won't work--and we are far more complex than a mouse trap.

Dr. Bill Bright, founder of Campus Crusade for Christ, spoke with scores of atheists on a one-to-one basis. Most initially conveyed the idea that they were unable to believe in such a book of myths or contradictions, but on closer questioning, revealed serious ignorance of basic Bible information.

<u>The bottom line for most of them</u> was, they were unprepared to accept the moral obligations that belief in the God of the Bible would require. A great theologian once said, "A man's morality dictates his theology."

Consider, for example, the Equidistant Lettering Sequences [ELS]. From the 1st yod in the 1st word of the Bible, "In the beginning, God created the heavens and the earth," (Genesis 1:1), counting every 521 letters spells "Yahshua yakhol" which means, "He is able" or has the power!

"Yahshua" is similarly encoded in dozens of Messianic prophecies. In Isaiah 53 where Christ "is brought as a lamb to the slaughter and taken from prison and from judgment," two verses later "he shall prolong his days" beginning with the 2nd yod, every 20 letters spells Yahshua Shmi--Yahshua is my name. *"Yeshua"* Yacov Rambsel, Frontier Research Publ.

Such design would not likely have been discovered until computers could search for the name and the message associated with it. But millions of people do not have computers; understanding such design is limited to few.

Nevertheless, the Bible in its plain text offers examples of encoding and complexity. Let the reader scan the information on the following webpage before clicking a particular link: http://www.pathlights.com/

Two atheist physicians had a complete change of mind, heart and medical practice by reading one of the finest books on health and happiness that I've found. You can read it free online, https://bit.ly/2kfpSfG

As a physician who was board-certified in internal medicine, I can tell you that the entire book is scientifically supported by the best of modern authorities.

193

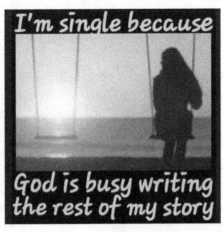

I'm single because

God is busy writing the rest of my story

Singles: Finding the Right Person to Marry

A young couple asked a pastor to marry them, but the girl's parents did not want them to marry. They said he was not right for their daughter. They appealed to the pastor for help.

He met with the couple and said he would marry them if they would spend a week talking about anything they wanted to talk about each evening, but no hugging or kissing.

A couple days later the girl called to say, 'He is the biggest bore I've ever met!' The wedding was off. She had been misled by affection that human nature likes.

Too many think they love each other because of physical affection, but that should only be the frosting on the cake of a good relationship that communicates well with each other.

Focus on the Family said 1st century marriages were contracted when a man and his son would visit another home of a man and his daughter.

The men would talk about the dowry price and the couple might be talking for the first time. They probably talked about everything--work, family, money, sex, religion, children, etc.

If the conversations were both agreeable, the father would give his son a cup of grape juice. He would offer it to the young lady saying, "This is my blood--I would shed it for you." If she accepted and drank from the cup, they were officially engaged.

He went home to build a room on his father's house and she would sew and get ready for his return in about a year for the wedding.

The key to happiness involves a mutual asking of wise questions and honesty in answering, but it was not clouded by physical affection that often misleads people today.

Sex may be the frosting on the cake of a good relationship, but many people only have frosting and soon they get sick...

A woman observed that many men play at love to get sex and many women play at sex to get love, and at the end of the game, the woman loses. Actually I think they both lose.

After my wife died from a prescription (explained in the chapter on health) I joined a Christian Singles Dating site. Those that I talked to wanted me to move nearby to get acquainted.

Moving was costly and risky if she wasn't the right person, so I asked them, Do you want a biblical marriage?

After explaining the information on 1st century marriages, most weren't so sure. Several wanted the "dating" process. But one woman was brave enough to talk the issues and we had lots in common that included food allergies--I'm blessed with a loving wife who's an excellent cook of foods that I can eat and it's been happy for nearly ten years.

As a further help to singles, it is usually the man's role to initiate things, and a woman should not dress in a way that is tempting to lustful thoughts.

Neat, and clean with modesty is a biblical principle, and not forward. On the other hand, Naomi's counsel to Ruth re Boaz seems forward but we don't know the customs then.

If single, pray and ask God to lead. The wives of Isaac, Jacob and Moses came from the well--they were taking care of sheep.

Christ said, feed my sheep. Finding someone else with a similar interest in spiritual things is reassuring.

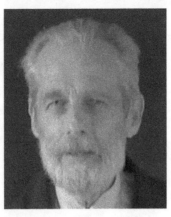

About the Author

Dr. Richard Ruhling is a retired physician who was board-certified in Internal Medicine and had a Cardiology Fellowship before teaching Health Science at Loma Linda University.

He attended cardiology meetings and was influenced by studies that showed heart disease could be reversed by diet. He says, We are what we eat and the good news is that we can reverse most disease as he explains in his NEW START seminar that features Nutrition, Exercise, Water Sunlight, Temperance, Air, Rest & Trust in God.

A Blue Cross manager brought his wife to the series and said it's the best he had seen in the wellness area that he worked so much with. The letter and sample video is on his speaker page at http://richardruhling.com/speaker.aspx

Media may contact Dr. Ruhling for interviews on book topics such as the coming war with Iran. Daniel's vision is "at th e time of the end," Daniel 8:17,20 names Persia (Iran). For a seminar at your church/group, please call **928 583 7543** or email him at Ruhling7@juno.com

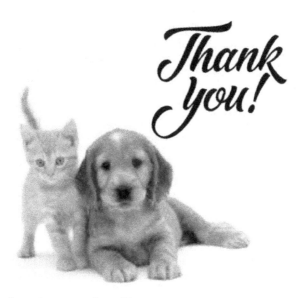

Websites that may be of interest

http://TheBridegroomComes.com

http://ChooseABetterDestiny.com

http://News4Living.wordpress.com

http://RichardRuhling.com/donate.aspx has the dvd and other books that you'll want to consider.

http://IslamUSinProphecy.wordpress.com

http://TheBridegroomComes.wordpress.com

http://LeadingCauseOfDeathPrescriptionDrugs.com

Cardiologist, Dr. Caldwell Esselstyn, https://bit.ly/2lVEQYz

Prof. of Nutrition, Dr. Colin Campbell, https://bit.ly/2kfm6Tz

Dr. Michael Gregor on numerous topics, https://bit.ly/2krtyuy

Dr. Daniel Amen on Brain Health, https://bit.ly/2koCpxf

Dr. Neal Barnard on Diabetes, https://bit.ly/2ltyK1s

Videos on Food Allergy, https://bit.ly/2jZFkfJ

PS Did you like this book? Whether it's the info above on prescription drugs or the chapter on singles, this book is packed with life-saving or life-changing information and it also shows how we can be part of the "Bride of Christ."

In Matthew 22:2, the King makes a marriage for His Son and He sends His servants to bid others to a wedding feast. We can be His servants and should want others to know how it can happen for them.

Please invite them to visit http://richardruhling.com For the price of a meal on the Donation page, they can have get this book *and The Earthquake & the 7 Seals* for just $5--it's Option 6.

The Earthquake & 7 Seals is the sequel to this and it's like the extra oil that wise virgins added to their lambs when the cry at midnight meant the Bridegroom is coming.

As Abraham Lincoln said, "I will study and get ready, and someday my chance will come." We should do the same by becoming familiar with Bible truths that God wants to have restored.

May God bless and guide you, and as Zig Ziglar, a Christian motivational speaker would say, "I'll see you at the Top!"

CPSIA information can be obtained
at www.ICGtesting.com
Printed in the USA
LVHW091519151121
703386LV00007B/442